Super Easy Carnivore Diet Cookbook

Effortless, High-Protein, Low-Carb Recipes for Meat Lovers - Delicious, Healthy, and Time-Saving Meals to Boost Your Energy & Shed Pounds!

Joshua Michael Davis

Table of Contents

Introduction to the Carnivore Diet

Imagine a diet so simple, yet so transformative, that it strips away the complexities of modern nutrition and takes you back to the basics—pure, unadulterated animal products.

The carnivore diet provides simplicity and clarity in a world where dietary recommendations are sometimes unclear and contradicting. It's not just a diet; it's a lifestyle that promises to revitalize your health, sharpen your mind, and energize your body. Whether you're seeking to shed stubborn pounds, reduce inflammation, or enhance your overall well-being, this cookbook is your gateway to discovering the incredible benefits of a meat-centric diet.

Inside, you'll find plenty mouth-watering recipes that celebrate the rich, savory flavors of meat in all its forms. From hearty breakfasts and tantalizing starters to sumptuous main dishes and decadent desserts, each recipe is crafted to nourish your body and delight your senses. This is not just about eating; it's about thriving.

So, are you ready to enjoy the power of meat and transform your health? Dive into the "Carnivore Diet Cookbook" and embark on a culinary journey that will change the way you think about food forever. Let's reclaim our health, one delicious bite at a time.

In recent years, the landscape of diet and nutrition has become increasingly diverse, with numerous plans promising health benefits and weight loss. From the Mediterranean diet, rich in grains, vegetables, and healthy fats, to the vegetarian and vegan diets that eliminate meat and animal products entirely, each offers unique advantages and challenges. Among these, the ketogenic diet restricts carbohydrates to leverage fats for energy, while the Paleo diet aims to mimic the eating habits of our hunter-gatherer ancestors. However, none is as extreme or straightforward as the carnivore diet, which demands a near-exclusive consumption of animal products.

The carnivore diet stands out due to its simplicity and radical approach. It eliminates all carbohydrates, including fruits and vegetables, focusing solely on meat, eggs, butter, and cheese. This diet harkens back to the dietary patterns of early humans, who often relied heavily on meat due to the scarcity and energy expenditure involved in gathering plant-based foods. While the carnivore diet might seem extreme in modern times, various cultures have historically thrived on similar dietary patterns, consuming predominantly animal-based products.

Despite its benefits, the carnivore diet is not for everyone. Pregnant women and children should avoid this diet to ensure they receive a broad spectrum of nutrients necessary for growth and development. For healthy adults, however, the carnivore diet can offer significant health improvements and weight loss.

To appreciate the distinctiveness of the carnivore diet, it's essential to understand the landscape of contemporary dietary practices. Popular diets like the Mediterranean, vegetarian, vegan, ketogenic, and Paleo diets each offer unique perspectives on what constitutes a healthy diet.

The Mediterranean diet, well-known for its heart-healthy advantages, places a strong emphasis on whole grains, fruits, and vegetables as well as healthy fats like olive oil. Fish and poultry should be consumed in moderation. Because of its high fiber and antioxidant content, it supports general health and lifespan.

Meat is excluded from vegetarian and vegan diets; vegans also abstain from all animal products, such as dairy and eggs. These diets are praised for their environmental benefits and potential to reduce the risk of chronic diseases. They are high in fiber, vitamins, and minerals, but they require careful planning to ensure adequate intake of essential nutrients like B12, iron, and protein.

The ketogenic diet is a low-carb, high-fat regimen designed to shift the body into a state of ketosis, where it burns fat for fuel instead of carbohydrates. It has shown promise in weight loss and management of certain neurological disorders but can be challenging to maintain long-term due to its restrictive nature.

Eating foods that are thought to have been available to people during the Paleolithic epoch is the main focus of paleo diets. This excludes processed foods, cereals, and dairy products and includes lean meats, fish, fruits, vegetables, nuts, and seeds. The goal is to mimic the eating habits of our ancestors, which proponents believe is more aligned with our genetic makeup.

Amid these diverse dietary philosophies, the carnivore diet emerges as a minimalist, almost primal approach. The carnivore diet is fundamentally just what it sounds like—a diet limited to foods derived from animals. This means meat, fish, eggs, and some dairy products form the entirety of one's diet, with a strict exclusion of all plant-based foods, including fruits, vegetables, grains, legumes, nuts, and seeds.

According to the carnivore diet, humans are meant to survive on a diet primarily consisting of animal fat and meat. Proponents argue that many of the health issues plaguing modern society, such as obesity, diabetes, and autoimmune diseases, can be attributed to the consumption of plant-based foods, particularly processed carbohydrates and sugars. By eliminating these from the diet, the carnivore approach aims to restore health and vitality.

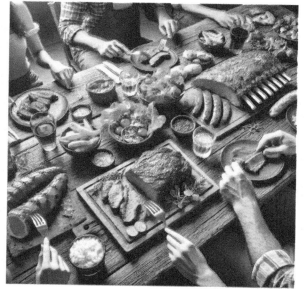

Historical Context and Evolutionary Perspective

To understand the rationale behind the carnivore diet, it's helpful to look at it through the lens of evolutionary biology. Our ancestors, long before the advent of agriculture, were hunter-gatherers. Their diets were largely dictated by the availability of food sources in their environment, which, for many, meant a diet rich in animal products.

During the Ice Age, for instance, plant foods were scarce, and early humans relied heavily on the animals they hunted. These ancient diets were high in protein and fat, with negligible carbohydrates. This period of human history suggests that our bodies are well-adapted to processing and thriving on meat-heavy diets.

Anthropological evidence points to various indigenous populations who have subsisted on predominantly animal-based diets for generations. The Inuit of the Arctic, the Maasai of East Africa, and certain Siberian tribes are often cited as examples. These groups have traditionally consumed diets high in animal fat and protein, with minimal plant intake, and have maintained excellent health without the chronic diseases prevalent in Western societies.

However, it's crucial to note that while these examples provide some support for the carnivore diet, they also highlight the importance of context. The specific environmental conditions, lifestyle, and genetic adaptations of these populations play a significant role in their dietary success. Translating these ancient or indigenous eating patterns to modern, diverse populations requires careful consideration and more scientific research.

The Rise of the Carnivore Diet

The carnivore diet's resurgence in recent years can be largely attributed to the growing disillusionment with conventional dietary guidelines and the rising popularity of low-carb, high-fat diets. Many individuals have found success with ketogenic diets, and the carnivore diet is seen as an extension of this, taking the low-carb concept to its extreme.

Prominent figures in the health and fitness community have also championed the carnivore diet, sharing personal anecdotes of dramatic weight loss, improved mental clarity, and relief from chronic health issues. These testimonials, often shared on social media platforms, have created a groundswell of interest and experimentation.

Dr. Shawn Baker, an orthopedic surgeon and one of the most vocal advocates of the carnivore diet, has played a pivotal role in popularizing this eating pattern. His book, "The Carnivore Diet," and numerous podcast appearances and interviews have helped bring the diet into the mainstream consciousness.

The Simplicity and Appeal of the Carnivore Diet

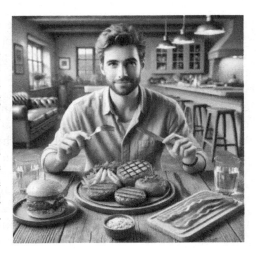

One of the most compelling aspects of the carnivore diet is its simplicity. In a world where dietary advice can often feel overwhelming and contradictory, the carnivore diet offers a straightforward solution: eat meat. This elimination of all plant-based foods simplifies meal planning and decision-making, reducing the cognitive load associated with maintaining a diet.

Moreover, the carnivore diet appeals to those who enjoy eating meat and are looking for a way to lose weight and improve their health without the need for extensive meal preparation or calorie counting. For many, the idea of eating hearty, satisfying meals composed of steaks, burgers, and bacon is far more appealing than a diet filled with salads and smoothies.

Scientific Scrutiny and Skepticism

Despite its growing popularity, the carnivore diet is not without controversy. Regarding its long-term health ramifications, scientists are still at odds. Some who argue against an all-meat diet claim that it is deficient in important nutrients including fiber, vitamins C and K, and several phytonutrients that are present in plant-based diets. There are concerns about the potential for nutrient deficiencies and the impact of high saturated fat intake on cardiovascular health.

Furthermore, it is challenging to reach firm conclusions regarding the safety and effectiveness of the carnivore diet due to the lack of long-term studies on its effects. Although preliminary studies and anecdotal evidence point to possible advantages, more thorough scientific investigation is required to support these assertions and determine the diet's long-term effects.

The carnivore diet offers a straightforward but contentious approach to nutrition, marking a dramatic break from accepted nutritional theory. Rooted in historical eating patterns and evolutionary biology, it challenges modern dietary norms and promises various health benefits. As with any diet, it is essential to approach the carnivore diet with a critical mind, considering individual health needs and consulting healthcare professionals before making significant dietary changes.

In the following sections, we will delve deeper into the specific benefits of the carnivore diet, address common questions and concerns, and provide practical steps for those interested in trying this unique dietary approach. Whether you are seeking weight loss, improved health, or simply a new perspective on eating, the carnivore diet offers a fascinating journey into the world of nutrition.

Benefits of the Carnivore Diet

The carnivore diet, a nutritional plan that centers around consuming only animal-based products, has been gaining traction in recent years. As radical as it might sound in today's carb-dominated world, the diet offers several compelling benefits that warrant a closer look. Let's delve into the key advantages that make the carnivore diet a potentially transformative approach to health and wellness.

Weight Management and Weight Loss

One of the most significant benefits of the carnivore diet is its effectiveness in managing and reducing body weight. By eliminating carbohydrates, the diet forces the body into a state of ketosis. Ketosis is a metabolic state where the body burns fat for fuel instead of carbohydrates, leading to substantial fat loss. This process is not only efficient for weight loss but also helps in maintaining a healthy weight over time.

The carnivore diet is inherently satiating due to its high protein and fat content. Because of their ability to keep you fuller for longer, these macronutrients can help you avoid overindulging and between-meal snacking. This natural reduction in calorie intake, combined with the increased fat-burning capacity of ketosis, makes weight loss almost effortless for many adherents.

Decreasing Inflammation

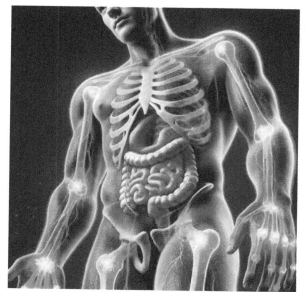

Chronic inflammation is a root cause of numerous health issues, including autoimmune diseases, cardiovascular diseases, and even cancer. Modern diets high in processed foods and sugars are known to exacerbate inflammatory responses in the body. The carnivore diet, however, is extremely low in carbohydrates and free from inflammatory foods like grains, legumes, and refined sugars.

By focusing on nutrient-dense animal products, which are naturally anti-inflammatory, the carnivore diet helps reduce inflammation. Omega-3 fatty acids, abundant in fatty fish and grass-fed meats, play a crucial role in combating inflammation. This reduction in inflammation can lead to noticeable improvements in conditions such as arthritis, irritable bowel syndrome (IBS), and other inflammatory diseases.

Increased Testosterone

For men, one of the notable benefits of the carnivore diet is the potential increase in testosterone levels. Testosterone is essential for muscle growth, bone density, brain function, and overall mood. Diets high in healthy fats and proteins, like the carnivore diet, support the production of testosterone, which can enhance physical performance, mental clarity, and general well-being.

Even women can benefit from balanced testosterone levels, which are important for muscle maintenance, libido, and mood regulation. The nutrient-rich profile of the carnivore diet, particularly from organ meats, provides the necessary building blocks for hormone production and balance.

Decreased Sugar Levels

The carnivore diet's strict elimination of all carbohydrates results in the absence of dietary sugars. Numerous health issues, such as obesity, diabetes, heart disease, and metabolic syndrome, are associated with high sugar intake. By cutting out sugar, the carnivore diet helps stabilize blood glucose levels, reducing the risk of insulin resistance and type 2 diabetes.

Stable blood sugar levels lead to fewer energy crashes and more constant energy throughout the day. This can lead to improved mental focus and productivity, making the carnivore diet particularly appealing for those with demanding lifestyles.

Reversing Insulin Resistance

Insulin resistance is a condition where the body's cells become less responsive to insulin, leading to higher blood sugar levels and increased fat storage. It is a precursor to type 2 diabetes and has been linked to a number of other health conditions, including heart disease and obesity.

The carnivore diet can help reverse insulin resistance by drastically reducing carbohydrate intake. This reduction lowers blood sugar levels and decreases the need for insulin, allowing the body's cells to regain their sensitivity to this crucial hormone. Over time, this can lead to improved blood sugar control and a reduced risk of developing diabetes and other metabolic disorders.

Increased Nutrient Density

Animal products, especially organ meats, are incredibly nutrient-dense. They contain a high concentration of important vitamins and minerals, which are typically deficient in modern diets.y. For instance, the liver is packed with vitamin A, vitamin B12, iron, and folate, all of which are vital for maintaining optimal health.

The carnivore diet ensures that you get a high intake of these critical nutrients without the need for supplementation. This nutrient density supports various bodily functions, including immune system strength, brain health, and overall vitality. The diet's focus on high-quality, unprocessed animal products ensures that you are consuming nutrients in their most bioavailable form.

Simplicity of the Diet

One of the major draws of the carnivore diet is its simplicity. In a world where diet plans can become overwhelmingly complex with calorie counting, portion control, and macronutrient tracking, the carnivore diet offers a refreshingly straightforward approach: eat animal products and avoid everything else.

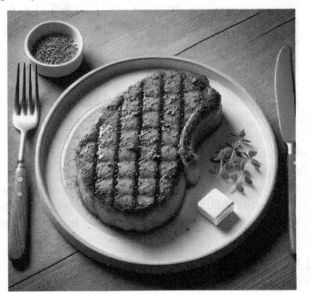

This simplicity makes it easier to follow and stick to the diet. There's no need to plan elaborate meals or track every bite you take. The clear, uncomplicated rules of the carnivore diet can help reduce the mental load associated with dietary changes, making it a sustainable long-term option for many people.

The carnivore diet presents a host of benefits that can significantly improve health and well-being. From effective weight management and reduction of chronic inflammation to increased testosterone and better blood sugar control, the diet addresses many of the common health challenges faced today. Its nutrient density ensures you receive essential vitamins and minerals, while its simplicity makes adherence straightforward and manageable.

The Carnivore Diet FAQ

As the carnivore diet continues to gain popularity, it's natural for people to have a multitude of questions. Whether you're a seasoned dieter or someone curious about this all-meat approach, understanding the fundamentals and addressing common concerns can help you make an informed decision. Here are some of the most frequently asked questions about the carnivore diet, answered.

How much fat and protein should I consume?

One of the first questions people have is about the macronutrient composition of the carnivore diet. The recommended ratio for most people is about 70-80% fat and 20-30% protein. This might seem counterintuitive, especially if you've been taught to avoid fat, but in the context of the carnivore diet, fat is your primary energy source.

For instance, if you consume 2000 calories a day, about 1400-1600 of those calories should come from fat (which translates to roughly 155-177 grams), and 400-600 calories from protein (approximately 100-150 grams). This balance allows your body to stay in ketosis, a state in which it uses fat for fuel rather than carbohydrates.

How Can I Increase My Fat Intake?

In a world where lean cuts of meat are often promoted, getting enough fat can be a challenge. However, there are several strategies you can use to boost your fat intake:

1. **Choose Fatty Cuts of Meat:** Opt for cuts like ribeye, pork belly, and fatty ground beef. These not only provide more fat but are also generally more flavorful.
2. **Add Butter:** Incorporating butter into your meals can significantly increase your fat intake. Use it to cook your meat, melt it over steaks, or even add a spoonful to your coffee.
3. **Eat More Fatty Fish:** Fish like salmon, mackerel, and sardines are excellent sources of healthy fats. They also provide beneficial omega-3 fatty acids.
4. **Use Animal Fats for Cooking:** Lard, tallow, and duck fat are great for cooking and add delicious flavor to your dishes.

How Many Meals Should I Eat Per Day?

One of the beauties of the carnivore diet is its flexibility. While the standard three meals a day works for some, many find that two meals a day, or even one large meal, suffices. The high protein and fat content of the diet means you'll feel fuller for longer, reducing the need for frequent meals.

It's also perfectly acceptable to listen to your body and eat when you're hungry. The satiety provided by the diet's macronutrient profile means you can trust your hunger signals more reliably than on a high-carb diet.

Will I Gain Muscle on This Diet?

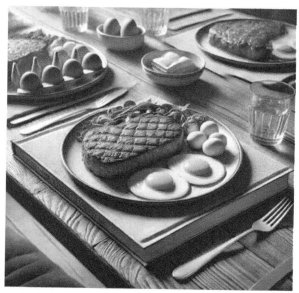

Absolutely. The carnivore diet is high in protein, which is essential for muscle repair and growth. Coupled with the fact that dietary fat helps boost testosterone levels, the diet can be particularly effective for those looking to gain muscle mass.

However, it's important to pair your diet with regular strength training to see significant muscle gains. The protein will provide the building blocks for muscle, while the fat ensures you have enough energy for intense workouts.

How Much Weight Will I Lose?

Weight reduction varies greatly from person to person and is determined by a number of factors, including initial weight, metabolic health, and adherence to the diet. Many people report losing 5-10 pounds in the first week, largely due to water weight loss as the body depletes its glycogen stores.

After the initial drop, weight loss typically continues at a slower, steady pace. Consuming fewer calories than you burn is essential for weight loss, and the satiating nature of the carnivore diet often makes this easier to achieve.

How long will it be until I adjust to this diet?

Adjusting to the carnivore diet can take time, especially if you're transitioning from a high-carb diet. Most people experience an adaptation period, sometimes referred to as the "keto flu," which can include symptoms like headaches, fatigue, and irritability. This typically lasts about 1-2 weeks.

To ease this transition, ensure you're drinking plenty of water and consider increasing your salt intake to balance electrolytes. Once your body adapts, you'll likely notice increased energy levels and improved overall well-being.

What About Fiber?

A common concern with the carnivore diet is the lack of fiber, traditionally thought to be essential for digestive health. Interestingly, many carnivore dieters report improved digestion and relief from conditions like IBS without any fiber intake.

Meat is efficiently digested in the stomach, and the elimination of plant fibers can reduce gut irritation for some individuals. If you experience digestive issues initially, give your body time to adapt. Most people find their digestion normalizes after a few weeks on the diet.

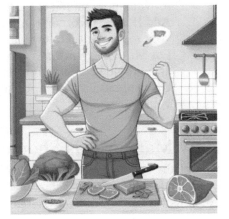

Is the Carnivore Diet Safe Long-Term?

Safety is a valid concern with any restrictive diet. While the long-term effects of the carnivore diet are still being studied, many people, including doctors and nutritionists who practice the diet themselves, report significant health benefits.

Key to long-term success is ensuring you consume a variety of animal products to get a broad spectrum of nutrients. This includes muscle meats, organ meats, and fish. Consulting with a healthcare provider before starting the diet can also help address any personal health concerns.

Can I Drink Coffee or Alcohol?

Coffee, particularly black coffee, is generally accepted on the carnivore diet as it contains no carbs or sugars. Many people find that it doesn't disrupt their ketosis and can even provide a welcomed boost of energy.

Alcohol, however, is more contentious. Most alcoholic beverages contain sugars and carbs, which are best avoided. If you choose to drink, stick to low-carb options like spirits (vodka, gin, whiskey) and avoid mixers that contain sugar. Always remember that alcohol can impair judgment, leading to poor dietary choices.

Do I Need Supplements?

While the carnivore diet can provide most of the nutrients your body needs, there are a few supplements that some people find beneficial:

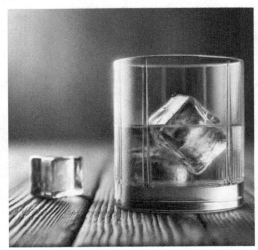

1. **Electrolytes:** During the initial adaptation phase, supplements for sodium, potassium, and magnesium can help mitigate "keto flu" symptoms.
2. **Omega-3s:** If you don't eat fatty fish frequently, an omega-3 supplement can help balance your fatty acid profile.
3. **Vitamin D:** Depending on your exposure to sunlight, a vitamin D supplement may be necessary, particularly in the winter months.

Can the Carnivore Diet Improve Mental Health?

Many adherents of the carnivore diet report significant improvements in mental clarity, mood, and overall mental health. The stabilization of blood sugar levels and the anti-inflammatory effects of the diet can contribute to these benefits.

Additionally, the elimination of dietary triggers like gluten and processed sugars, which can impact mood and cognitive function, may lead to enhanced mental well-being.

Steps to Get Started on the Carnivore Diet

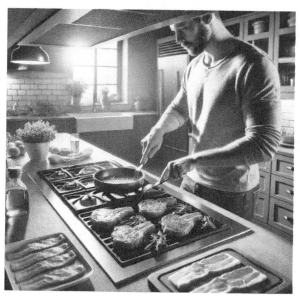

Embarking on the carnivore diet is a transformative journey that can lead to significant health benefits and an improved quality of life. To achieve success, however, it is necessary to prepare carefully and follow a disciplined approach, as with any major lifestyle adjustment. Here are the key steps to get started on the carnivore diet, presented in a way that makes the transition as smooth and sustainable as possible.

Step 1: Exercise & Liquid Calorie Removal

Before you dive into the carnivore diet, it's essential to start with a clean slate. This means eliminating all liquid calories from your diet. Beverages like sugary sodas, fruit juices, and even many flavored waters are packed with unnecessary sugars and calories that can sabotage your progress. Switch to unsweetened tea, black coffee, and, most importantly, water.

Simultaneously, begin incorporating some form of exercise into your routine. You don't need to become a gym rat overnight, but adding a daily 30-minute walk can do wonders for your overall health and help your body transition to the new diet. Physical activity helps to boost your metabolism and aids in the efficient utilization of nutrients.

Step 2: Get Rid of Junk Food

The next crucial step is to purge your kitchen of all junk food. This includes sugary snacks, processed foods, and any items that do not fit within the carnivore diet's strict guidelines. It's easier to avoid temptation when these foods are simply not available.

To make this transition smoother, do it gradually over a week. Start by eliminating the obvious culprits like candy, chips, and soda. Then, move on to more subtle sources of carbs and sugars, such as cereals, granola bars, and even some seemingly healthy snacks that are laden with hidden sugars and grains. The goal is to create an environment that supports your new dietary commitment.

Step 3: Remove Grains, Legumes, and Cereals

Grains, legumes, and cereals are staples in many diets, but they have no place in the carnivore diet. These foods are high in carbohydrates and can cause inflammation and digestive issues for some people. Begin by cutting out bread, pasta, rice, beans, lentils, and other grain-based products from your meals.

This step can be challenging, especially if you're used to having these foods as dietary mainstays. A good strategy is to find suitable replacements within the carnivore guidelines, such as enjoying a hearty steak or a satisfying portion of bacon and eggs. Focus on the delicious and filling options available to you.

Step 4: Reduce Carbs

After removing the primary sources of carbohydrates, it's time to reduce your overall carb intake. This involves cutting down on vegetables and fruits, which are typically encouraged in most other diets. While they offer vitamins and minerals, the carnivore diet posits that you can get all the nutrients you need from animal products.

Transitioning away from a high-carb diet to a low-carb diet can be a significant adjustment for your body. Take it slowly by gradually decreasing your carb intake over a few weeks. This method helps to minimize withdrawal symptoms like headaches, fatigue, and cravings.

Step 5: Use Intermittent Fasting

Intermittent fasting isn't a requirement for the carnivore diet, but it can be a helpful tool during the transition phase. Fasting helps to regulate your eating patterns and aligns with the natural cycles of hunger and satiety. The 16/8 method is a popular approach in which you fast for 16 hours and then eat all of your meals within an 8-hour timeframe.

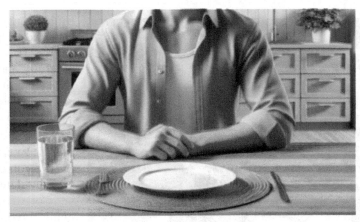

Intermittent fasting can help you get used to eating fewer meals and can support the metabolic shift to burning fat for fuel. Many people find that fasting becomes easier once they are fully adapted to the carnivore diet because the high protein and fat intake keeps them feeling full for longer periods.

Step 6: Cut Carbs Further

Once you're comfortable with a low-carb intake, it's time to cut carbs even further, aiming for less than 25 grams per day. This phase is important for achieving and maintaining ketosis, in which your body transforms into a fat-burning machine.

During this phase, you may want to experiment with ketogenic recipes that align closely with the carnivore diet. Focus on high-fat, moderate-protein meals that are satisfying and keep your carb intake minimal. Remember, the goal is to shift your body into a state where it primarily uses fat for energy.

Step 7: Remove Vegetables & Vegetable Oils

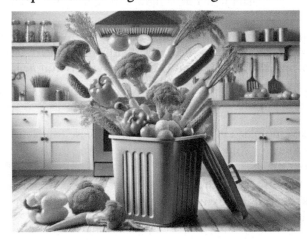

This step involves eliminating the last remnants of plant-based foods from your diet, including vegetables and vegetable oils. While vegetables are often considered healthy, they contain carbohydrates that can impede ketosis. Moreover, many vegetable oils are highly processed and can cause inflammation.

Replace vegetable oils with animal fats like butter, ghee, tallow, and lard. These fats not only align with the carnivore diet but also offer a rich flavor and a source of energy. Cooking with animal fats is not only healthier but also enhances the taste of your meals.

Step 8: Animal Products Only

The final step is fully committing to eating only animal products. This includes meat, fish, eggs, and dairy (if tolerated). At this stage, you should have a well-stocked pantry with a variety of animal-based foods to keep your meals interesting and enjoyable.

Focus on a variety of meats such as beef, pork, lamb, and poultry. Incorporate organ meats like liver, which are nutrient-dense and provide essential vitamins and minerals. Fish and seafood are also excellent choices, offering beneficial omega-3 fatty acids. If you tolerate dairy, include high-fat options like cheese and cream to add variety and richness to your diet.

Additional Tips for Success

- **Stay Hydrated:** Drinking enough of water is essential, especially during the early transition period. Adequate hydration helps to flush out toxins and can alleviate common symptoms like headaches and fatigue.

- **Listen to Your Body:** Monitor how your body reacts to the diet. Some people may need to make minor adjustments based on their unique nutritional needs and health conditions.

- **Plan Your Meals:** Planning your meals ahead of time can help you stay on track. Prepare larger portions and make use of leftovers to ensure you always have a carnivore-friendly meal ready.

- **Stay Patient:** Adapting to the carnivore diet can take time. It's normal to feel some discomfort until your body adjusts. Stay committed and give yourself time to adapt.

- **Seek Support:** Finding a community or a buddy who is also following the carnivore diet can provide motivation and support. Sharing experiences and tips can make the transition easier and more enjoyable.

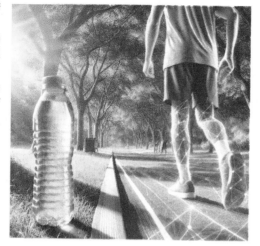

Your Shopping List

Embarking on the carnivore diet requires a thoughtful approach to grocery shopping. Since this diet focuses exclusively on animal products, it's essential to stock up on the right kinds of foods to ensure you're getting a variety of nutrients and enjoying your meals. Here's a comprehensive shopping list to get you started on your carnivorous journey.

Beef Go-To's

When it comes to the carnivore diet, beef should be a staple in your kitchen. Opt for fatty cuts to meet your nutritional needs and to keep your meals satisfying.

- **Ribeye Steaks**: These are not only delicious but also packed with fats and proteins.
- **Ground Beef**: Versatile and easy to cook, aim for 80/20 ground beef for a good fat-to-protein ratio.
- **Chuck Roast**: Great for slow-cooking, this cut is both flavorful and budget-friendly.
- **Short Ribs**: Perfect for braising or slow-cooking, providing a rich and hearty meal.
- **Beef Brisket**: Another excellent option for slow-cooking, yielding tender and juicy results.

Other Meats

While beef is a cornerstone, diversifying your meat intake can keep your meals interesting and nutritionally balanced.

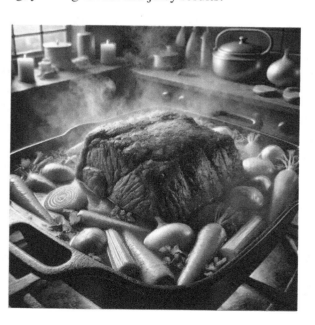

- **Pork**: Look for pork belly, shoulder, and ribs. These cuts are fatty and flavorful.
- **Lamb**: Lamb chops, shanks, and shoulder are great choices, offering a different taste profile.
- **Poultry**: Chicken thighs, drumsticks, and wings are preferable over breast meat due to their higher fat content. Duck is also a fantastic option.
- **Seafood**: Salmon, sardines, mackerel, and shrimp are excellent sources of omega-3 fatty acids. Shellfish like oysters and mussels are nutrient-dense and can add variety.
- **Organ Meats**: The liver, heart, and kidneys are nutrient dense. They might take some getting used to, but they're incredibly beneficial.

Beverages

On the carnivore diet, your beverage options are limited, but there are still a few to enjoy.

- **Water**: The most crucial beverage. Consider both still and sparkling varieties to keep things interesting.
- **Bone Broth**: Packed with nutrients, bone broth is excellent for sipping and adding to dishes.
- **Black Coffee**: If you can't give up your morning ritual, black coffee is acceptable.
- **Tea**: Unsweetened tea can also be included, providing a bit of variety.

Other Permissible Foods

While the carnivore diet is restrictive, there are a few additional items that can complement your meals.

- **Eggs**: A versatile and economical protein source, eggs are a household staple.
- **Butter and Ghee**: Essential for cooking and adding extra fat to your meals.
- **Cheese**: Opt for full-fat cheeses like cheddar, blue cheese, and cream cheese.
- **Seasonings**: Keep it simple with salt, pepper, and herbs like thyme and rosemary to enhance the flavor of your meats.

Tips & Tricks to Help

Transitioning to the carnivore diet can be challenging, but with the right strategies, you can make the switch smoothly and sustainably. Here are some expert tips and tricks to help you stay on track and enjoy the process.

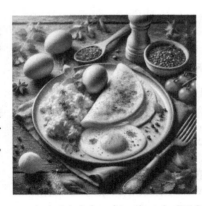

Eat Eggs

Eggs are an incredibly nutrient-dense food, providing essential vitamins and minerals. They are also versatile and easy to prepare. Incorporate eggs into your diet for variety and to boost your nutrient intake. Scramble them for breakfast, hard-boil them for snacks, or use them in recipes like frittatas and omelets.

Eat Liver (And Other Organs!)

Organ meats are some of the most nutritious foods you can consume. Liver, in instance, is high in vitamins A, B12, and iron. If you're not used to eating liver, start with small amounts and gradually increase your intake. You can also blend liver into ground beef dishes to make it more palatable.

Eat Seafood

Adding seafood to your diet can provide essential omega-3 fatty acids, which are important for heart health. Fatty seafood such as salmon, mackerel, and sardines are great options. Shellfish, such as oysters and mussels, are also incredibly nutrient-dense and offer a different flavor profile to keep your meals interesting.

Use Bone Broth

Bone broth is not only delicious but also packed with nutrients like collagen, amino acids, and minerals. It's great for gut health and can help reduce inflammation. Sip on bone broth as a warm drink or use it as a base for soups and stews.

Pick Your Schedule

Establishing a consistent eating schedule can help you stick to the carnivore diet more easily. Some people find success with intermittent fasting, eating all their meals within an 8-hour window. This method can help control your appetite. and support weight loss. However, find what works best for you, whether it's two meals a day or three smaller ones.

Eat Slowly

Taking your time when eating allows your body to detect when you're full, which helps prevent overeating. Eating slowly also enhances digestion and can make mealtimes more enjoyable. Concentrate on enjoying each bite and listening to your body's hunger cues.

Make Leftovers

Cooking in bulk and having leftovers can save time and make sticking to the diet easier. Prepare larger portions of meals and store them in the fridge or freezer for quick and easy access throughout the week. This approach minimizes the temptation to deviate from the diet due to lack of time or convenience.

Stay Hydrated

Staying hydrated is crucial on the carnivore diet. Drink plenty of water throughout the day to support digestion and overall health. If you find plain water boring, try sparkling water or add a splash of lemon juice for flavor. Bone broth can also contribute to your hydration needs.

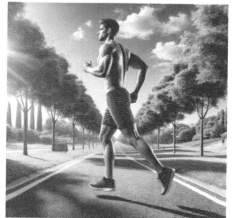

Add In Exercise

Incorporating regular exercise into your routine can enhance the benefits of the carnivore diet. Physical activity helps maintain muscle mass, supports metabolism, and improves overall well-being. To maintain your body's strength and health, combine strength training with cardiovascular exercises.

Grab A Buddy

Having a support system can significantly improve your success with the carnivorous diet. Find a friend or family member who is also interested in trying the diet and support each other through the process. Sharing recipes, tips, and experiences can make the journey more enjoyable and sustainable.

Introduction to Carnivore Diet Recipes

Transitioning to the carnivore diet can be a significant shift for many people, especially if you're used to a diverse diet that includes plenty of fruits, vegetables, and grains. One of the keys to success on this diet is not just understanding the nutritional science behind it but also having a wide array of delicious recipes at your disposal. This chapter is dedicated to introducing you to 120 mouth-watering carnivore recipes that will make your journey enjoyable and sustainable.

The Importance of Variety in the Carnivore Diet

While the carnivore diet is inherently restrictive, focusing solely on animal-based products, it doesn't have to be monotonous. Variety is essential not only for maintaining enthusiasm for your meals but also for ensuring you get a broad spectrum of nutrients. Each type of meat and animal product offers a unique nutrient profile, and experimenting with different cuts, preparation methods, and flavorings can help keep your palate excited.

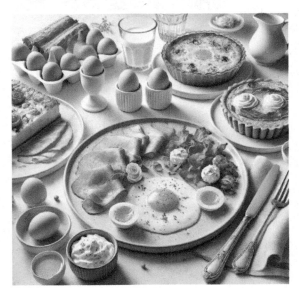

Navigating the World of Carnivore Recipes

The carnivore diet can initially seem daunting due to its limited food selection. However, the simplicity of the ingredients can be transformed into culinary creativity with the right recipes. This chapter will guide you through a variety of meal options, from quick and easy breakfasts to elaborate dinners, ensuring you never feel deprived or bored.

Breakfasts That Kickstart Your Day

Breakfast on the carnivore diet can be both satisfying and energizing. Eggs, a staple for many, can be prepared in numerous ways to keep things interesting. Think beyond the standard scrambled or fried eggs. Try out an egg and ham bake, goat cheese and ham frittata, or a bacon and egg quiche. These recipes are not only delicious but also packed with the fats and proteins needed to fuel your morning.

Hearty Lunches to Power Through Your Day

Lunches on the carnivore diet can be hearty and fulfilling. Imagine enjoying a grilled lamb coated in cumin, a ribeye steak with cheese sauce, or smoked mutton paired with roasted marrow. These meals are designed to be rich in flavor and nutrients, keeping you satisfied throughout the afternoon. Slow cooker recipes like pork shoulder or lamb shanks can be prepared in advance, making your midday meal both convenient and delectable.

Dinners That Delight

Dinners are where you can truly indulge in the rich, savory flavors of the carnivore diet. From a garlic bison rib roast to a slow-cooked beef brisket, the possibilities are endless. These recipes often involve longer cooking times and more complex preparation methods, resulting in deeply flavorful and tender dishes. Pair your main course with simple sides like roasted bone marrow or bacon-wrapped asparagus for a complete meal.

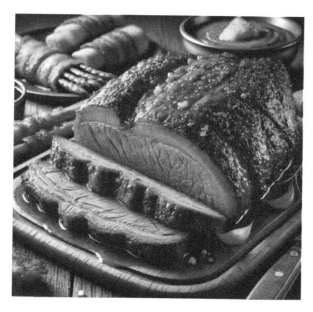

Exploring Seafood Options

Seafood is an excellent addition to the carnivore diet, offering variety and essential omega-3 fatty acids. Recipes such as garlic and cilantro salmon, roasted thyme swordfish, and creamy baked cod are not only easy to prepare but also elevate your meals with their unique flavors. Seafood can provide a refreshing change from red meat and poultry, ensuring your diet remains balanced and diverse.

Incorporating Organ Meats

Organ meats are some of the most nutrient-dense foods available, yet they are often overlooked. Recipes like Mediterranean liver steak, crispy tripe, and liver patties can introduce you to the health benefits and flavors of these powerful foods. While they might require an adjustment period, the nutritional advantages they offer make them a valuable addition to your diet.

Cooking Techniques for Maximum Flavor

The method you use to cook your food can greatly impact its flavor and texture. Here are some techniques to enhance your carnivore meals:

- **Grilling**: Adds a smoky flavor and creates a crispy exterior while keeping the inside juicy.
- **Slow cooking:** ideal for harder types of meat since it gradually softens and enhances their flavor.
- **Pan Searing**: Quickly cooks the meat at high temperatures, creating a delicious crust.
- **Roasting**: Ideal for larger cuts, providing a tender interior with a caramelized exterior.
- **Braising**: Combines dry and wet heat, perfect for infusing flavors into the meat.

Flavoring Your Meals

While the carnivore diet limits many traditional seasonings, you can still create flavorful dishes using animal-based products and a few approved seasonings. Salt, pepper, garlic, and herbs like rosemary and thyme can significantly enhance your meals. Additionally, using animal fats like butter and ghee for cooking adds depth and richness to your dishes.

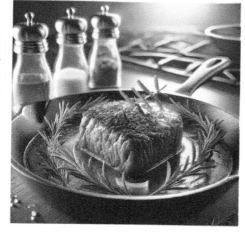

Tips for Success in Carnivore Cooking

To get the most out of your carnivore recipes, consider the following tips:

- **Quality Ingredients:** Always opt for high-quality, grass-fed, and pasture-raised meats when possible. The quality of your ingredients can make a significant difference in taste and nutritional value.
- **Meal Prep:** Arrange and cook your meals ahead of time. Cooking larger portions and having leftovers can save time and ensure you have delicious, carnivore-friendly meals ready to go.
- **Experimentation**: Don't be afraid to try new cuts of meat or cooking methods. Experimenting can help you discover new favorite recipes and keep your diet exciting.
- **Hydration**: Drink plenty of water and consider incorporating bone broth into your diet to stay hydrated and support your health.
- **Listen to Your Body**: Pay attention to how your body responds to different foods and adjust accordingly. Since each person has unique nutritional needs, it's critical to customize your diet to meet those needs.

Adapting Recipes to Your Preferences

One of the great things about the carnivore diet is its flexibility within its restrictions. Feel free to modify recipes to fit your dietary requirements and taste preferences. If you prefer certain meats or have access to specific ingredients, customize the recipes accordingly. The goal is to create meals that you enjoy and that support your health.

The carnivore diet offers a unique approach to nutrition that can be both satisfying and beneficial for your health. By incorporating a variety of recipes and cooking techniques, you can ensure that your meals are not only nutritious but also delicious. This chapter has introduced you to the world of carnivore cooking, providing you with the tools and inspiration to create enjoyable meals that keep you committed to your dietary goals.

As you explore the 120 recipes provided, remember that the key to success on the carnivore diet is finding what works best for you. Embrace the journey, experiment with new dishes, and enjoy the process of nourishing your body with high-quality, animal-based foods. With the right mindset and resources, you can thrive on the carnivore diet and reap its many benefits.

Carnivore Diet Recipes

Breakfast

Egg & Ham Bake

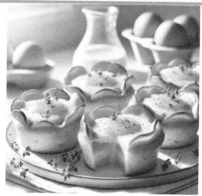

Ingredients:
- 6 large eggs
- 12 slices ham
- ½ cup heavy cream
- 1 tablespoon Dijon mustard
- 1 tablespoon fresh thyme, chopped
- Sea salt and black pepper to taste

Directions:
1. Preheat your oven to 370°F (190°C) and place the oven rack in the lowest slot.
2. Spray a muffin tray with cooking spray and place the ham slices in the cups, allowing them to flow over the sides.
3. In a large bowl, whisk together the eggs, heavy cream, Dijon mustard, thyme, sea salt, and black pepper until well combined.
4. Pour the egg mixture into the ham-lined cups, filling each about three-quarters full.
5. Bake for 10-15 minutes, or until the ham is crisp and the eggs are fully cooked. A toothpick inserted into the center should come out clean.
6. Allow the bakes to cool for 5 minutes before serving warm.

Number of servings: 6

Preparation time: 10 minutes

Cooking time: 45 minutes

Nutritional value per serving: Calories: 150, Carbs: 1g, Fiber: 0g, Sugars: 0g, Protein: 12g, Saturated fat: 5g, Unsaturated fat: 3g

Difficulty rating:
★★☆☆☆

Tips for ingredient variations: Add 1/4 cup shredded cheese of your choice to the egg mixture for a richer flavor.

Bacon & Cheddar Breakfast Muffins

Number of servings: 6

Preparation time: 15 minutes

Cooking time: 25 minutes

Nutritional value per serving: Calories: 230, Carbs: 1g, Fiber: 0g, Sugars: 0g, Protein: 12g, Saturated fat: 15g, Unsaturated fat: 5g

Difficulty rating:
★★☆☆☆

Tips for ingredient variations: Add finely chopped vegetables like bell peppers or spinach for added nutrition and flavor.

Directions:
1. Preheat your oven to 375° F (190° C).
2. Beat the eggs, heavy cream, salt, and pepper in a big bowl until thoroughly blended.
3. Melt the butter in a skillet over medium heat. Add the crumbled bacon and cook for 2 minutes.
4. Pour the egg mixture into the skillet and cook for 3-4 minutes, stirring occasionally, until slightly thickened.
5. Grease a muffin tin with butter or non-stick spray. Divide the egg mixture evenly among the muffin cups.
6. Sprinkle the shredded cheddar cheese evenly over the top of each muffin.
7. Bake in the preheated oven for 15 minutes, or until the muffins are firm and cooked through.
8. Before taking them out of the muffin tray, let them cool slightly. Serve warm

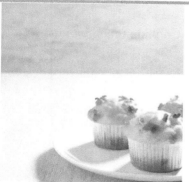

Ingredients:
- Sea salt and black pepper to taste
- 1 cup shredded cheddar cheese
- 6 slices of bacon, cooked and crumbled
- 2 tablespoons butter
- 8 large eggs
- 1/2 cup heavy cream

Sausage & Cheese Breakfast Casserole

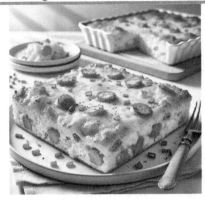

Ingredients:
- 8 large eggs
- 1 cup heavy cream
- 1 lb ground sausage
- 1 cup shredded cheddar cheese
- 1 cup shredded mozzarella cheese
- 1/2 cup grated Parmesan cheese
- 1/4 teaspoon garlic powder
- 1/4 teaspoon onion powder
- Sea salt and black pepper to taste
- 2 tablespoons fresh chives, chopped

Directions:
1. Preheat your oven to 350°F (175°C).
2. Cook the sausage to a brown texture in a pan over medium heat. Empty the extra fat.
3. In a large bowl, whisk together the eggs, heavy cream, garlic powder, onion powder, salt, and pepper.
4. Grease a 9x13 inch baking dish and spread the cooked sausage evenly across the bottom.
5. Pour the egg mixture over the sausage.
6. Sprinkle the shredded cheddar, mozzarella, and Parmesan cheeses evenly over the top.
7. Bake for 45 minutes, or until the casserole is set and the top is golden brown.
8. Before slicing, let the casserole cool for ten minutes. Garnish with chopped chives and serve warm.

Number of servings: 4

Preparation time: 20 minutes

Cooking time: 45 minutes

Nutritional value per serving: Calories: 620, Carbs: 4g, Fiber: 0g, Sugars: 1g, Protein: 38g, Saturated fat: 29g Unsaturated fat: 18g

Difficulty rating:
★★★☆☆

Tips for ingredient variations: For added flavor, mix in 1/2 cup of sautéed mushrooms or bell peppers into the sausage layer before adding the egg mixture.

Poached Eggs

Number of servings: 1

Preparation time: 5 minutes

Cooking time: 5 minutes

Nutritional value per serving: Calories: 230, Carbs: 1g, Fiber: 0g, Sugars: 0g, Protein: 13g, Saturated fat: 12g, Unsaturated fat: 6g

Difficulty rating: ★☆☆☆☆

Tips for ingredient variations: For an added flavor twist, sprinkle some freshly cracked black pepper or a pinch of paprika on top before serving.

Directions:
1. Heat a skillet over medium heat and melt the butter until it begins to sizzle.
2. Crack the eggs gently into the skillet, keeping the yolks intact.
3. Sprinkle the eggs with salt and cook until the whites are set but the yolks remain runny, about 3-4 minutes.
4. Carefully remove the eggs from the skillet using a spatula and serve warm.

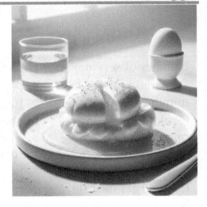

Ingredients:
- 2 large eggs
- ½ teaspoon salt
- 3 tablespoons butter

Scrambled Eggs with Butter

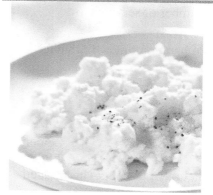

Ingredients:
- 4 large eggs
- 2 tablespoons butter
- Sea salt and black pepper to taste

Directions:
1. Crack the eggs into a mixing basin and whisk until the yolks and whites are well mixed.
2. Heat a non-stick skillet over medium-low heat and melt the butter.
3. Pour the eggs into the skillet and let them sit, without stirring, for about 1-2 minutes.
4. Gently whisk the eggs with a spatula, moving them from the borders to the middle, until they begin to curdle.
5. Continue cooking until the eggs are just set but still slightly creamy, about 2-3 minutes more.
6. Serve warm, seasoning with sea salt and black pepper to taste.

Number of servings: 2
Preparation time: 5 minutes
Cooking time: 5 minutes
Nutritional value per serving: Calories: 220, Carbs: 1g, Fiber: 0g, Sugars: 1g, Protein: 12g, Saturated fat: 12g, Unsaturated fat: 6g

Difficulty rating: ★☆☆☆

Tips for ingredient variations: Add a tablespoon of heavy cream to the eggs before whisking for extra creaminess.

Omelette with Cheddar Cheese

Number of servings: 1
Preparation time: 5 minutes
Cooking time: 10 minutes
Nutritional value per serving: Calories: 350, Carbs: 1g, Fiber: 0g, Sugars: 1g, Protein: 20g, Saturated fat: 22g, Unsaturated fat: 8g

Difficulty rating: ★★☆☆

Tips for ingredient variations: Add finely chopped chives or cooked bacon bits to the cheese before folding the omelet for an added flavor boost.

Directions:
1. Crack the eggs into a bowl and whisk until well combined.
2. Heat a non-stick skillet over medium heat and melt the butter.
3. Pour the eggs into the skillet, swirling to create an even layer.
4. Cook for two to three minutes, or until the edges begin to set, without stirring.
5. Sprinkle the cheddar cheese evenly over one half of the omelet.
6. Fold the omelet in half over the cheese and cook until the cheese is melted and the eggs are fully set, about 2-3 minutes more.
7. Serve warm, seasoned to taste with a pinch of sea salt and black pepper.

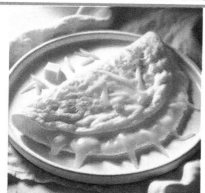

Ingredients:
- 3 large eggs
- 2 tablespoons butter
- 1/2 cup shredded cheddar cheese
- Sea salt and black pepper to taste

Soft-Boiled Eggs with Sea Salt

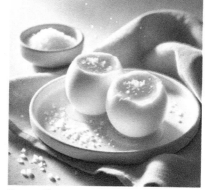

Ingredients:
- 2 large eggs
- ½ teaspoon sea salt

Directions:
1. Bring a pot of water to a gentle boil over medium-high heat.
2. Carefully lower the eggs into the boiling water using a spoon.
3. Boil the eggs for 6-7 minutes for a soft, runny yolk.
4. Remove the eggs from the boiling water and place them in a bowl of ice water for 1 minute to stop the cooking process.
5. Peel the eggs and sprinkle with sea salt before serving.

Number of servings: 1
Preparation time: 5 minutes
Cooking time: 7 minutes
Nutritional value per serving: Calories: 140, Carbs: 1g, Fiber: 0g, Sugars: 0g, Protein: 12g, Saturated fat: 3g, Unsaturated fat: 5g

Difficulty rating: ★☆☆☆

Tips for ingredient variations: Serve with a side of buttered, toasted carnivore bread for added texture and flavor.

Egg Muffins with Sausage

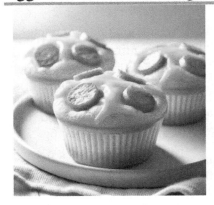

Ingredients:
• 8 large eggs
• 1 cup cooked sausage, crumbled
• ½ cup heavy cream
• 1 cup shredded cheddar cheese
Sea salt and black pepper to taste

Directions:
1. Preheat your oven to 375° F (190° C).
2. Use cooking spray to grease a muffin tray.
3. In a large bowl, whisk together the eggs, heavy cream, salt, and pepper.
4. Divide the cooked sausage and shredded cheese evenly among the muffin cups.
5. Pour the egg mixture over the sausage and cheese, filling each cup about three-quarters full.
6. Bake the egg muffins for 20 to 25 minutes, or until they are firm and have a hint of color on top.
7. Allow the muffins to cool for 5 minutes before removing from the tin. Serve warm.

Number of servings: 6

Preparation time: 10 minutes

Cooking time: 25 minutes

Nutritional value per serving:
Calories: 280, Carbs: 2g, Fiber: 0g, Sugars: 0g, Protein: 20g, Saturated fat: 16g, Unsaturated fat: 6g

Difficulty rating: ★★☆☆

Tips for ingredient variations: Add chopped bell peppers or spinach for extra flavor and nutrients.

Carnivore Pancakes (Egg and Pork Rinds)

Number of servings: 2

Preparation time: 5 minutes

Cooking time: 10 minutes

Nutritional value per serving: Calories: 340, Carbs: 1g, Fiber: 0g, Sugars: 0g, Protein: 20g, Saturated fat: 16g, Unsaturated fat: 6g

Difficulty rating: ★★☆☆

Tips for ingredient variations: For a sweeter version, add a few drops of liquid stevia or a sprinkle of cinnamon to the batter.

Directions:
1. In a blender, combine the eggs, crushed pork rinds, heavy cream, and vanilla extract. Blend until smooth.
2. Heat a non-stick skillet over medium heat and melt the butter.
3. Pour the batter into the skillet to form small pancakes, cooking in batches if necessary.
4. Cook for 2-3 minutes on each side, or until the pancakes are golden brown and cooked through.
5. Serve warm with additional butter or a drizzle of heavy cream if desired.

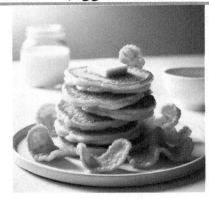

Ingredients:
• 4 large eggs
• ½ cup pork rinds, crushed
• ¼ cup heavy cream
• 1 teaspoon vanilla extract
1 tablespoon butter (for cooking)

Steak and Eggs

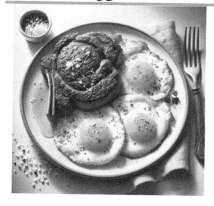

Ingredients:

• 2 ribeye steaks (about 8 oz each)
• 4 large eggs
• 2 tablespoons butter
• Sea salt and black pepper to taste
• 1 tablespoon fresh parsley, chopped (optional)

Directions:

1. Preheat a skillet over medium-high heat and add 1 tablespoon of butter.
2. Season the steaks with sea salt and black pepper.
3. Cook the steaks in the skillet for 4-5 minutes per side, or until they reach your desired level of doneness. Remove from the skillet and let them rest.
4. In the same skillet, add the remaining 1 tablespoon of butter.
5. Once the eggs are cracked into the skillet, fry them to your desired consistency (over-easy, sunny-side up, etc.).
6. Serve the eggs alongside the steaks. Sprinkle with fresh parsley if desired.

Number of servings: 2

Preparation time: 10 minutes

Cooking time: 15 minutes

Nutritional value per serving: Calories: 650, Carbs: 1g, Fiber: 0g, Sugars: 0g, Protein: 48g, Saturated fat: 25g, Unsaturated fat: 20g

Difficulty rating: ★★☆☆

Tips for ingredient variations: Add a side of sautéed mushrooms or spinach for extra flavor and nutrients.

Eggs Benedict with Hollandaise Sauce

Number of servings: 4

Preparation time: 15 minutes

Cooking time: 20 minutes

Nutritional value per serving: Calories: 400, Carbs: 1g, Fiber: 0g, Sugars: 0g, Protein: 20g, Saturated fat: 30g, Unsaturated fat: 10g

Difficulty rating: ★★★★☆

Tips for ingredient variations: Add a sprinkle of smoked paprika or cayenne pepper to the hollandaise sauce for a spicy kick.

Directions:

1. To make the hollandaise sauce, whisk the egg yolks and lemon juice in a heatproof bowl over a pot of simmering water. Slowly add the melted butter while continuously whisking until the sauce thickens. Season with sea salt and set aside.
2. In a skillet, melt 2 tablespoons of butter over medium heat and cook the ham slices until lightly browned. Remove from the skillet and keep warm.
3. Fill a large saucepan with water and bring to a gentle simmer. Add a dash of vinegar and a bit of salt (optional). Once the eggs are cracked into the water, poach them for three to four minutes, or until the yolks are still runny but the whites are set.
4. To assemble, put a poached egg on top of a slice of ham on each plate, then pour hollandaise sauce over it. Season with salt and pepper.
5. Serve immediately.

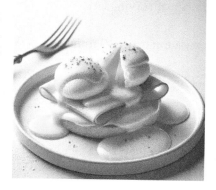

Ingredients:

• 8 large eggs
• 4 slices ham
• 4 tablespoons butter, divided
• Sea salt and black pepper to taste
Hollandaise Sauce:
• 3 egg yolks
• 1 tablespoon lemon juice
• 1/2 cup melted butter
• Sea salt to taste

Carnivore Breakfast Pizza (Eggs, Bacon, Cheese)

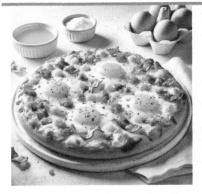

Ingredients:

• 6 large eggs
• 1 cup shredded cheese (cheddar, mozzarella, or your choice)
• 6 slices bacon, cooked and crumbled
• Sea salt and black pepper to taste
• 2 tablespoons butter

Directions:

1. Preheat your oven to 375° F (190° C).

2. In a large bowl, whisk together the eggs and season with sea salt and black pepper.

3. In a large oven-safe skillet, melt the butter over medium heat.

4. Pour the egg mixture into the skillet and cook for 2-3 minutes, until the edges start to set.

5. Sprinkle the shredded cheese evenly over the eggs, followed by the crumbled bacon.

6. After placing the pan in the oven, bake it for ten to fifteen minutes, or until the cheese has melted and become bubbling and the eggs are set.

Slice and serve warm.

Number of servings: 4

Preparation time: 10 minutes

Cooking time: 20 minutes

Nutritional value per serving: Calories: 300, Carbs: 1g, Fiber: 0g, Sugars: 0g, Protein: 22g, Saturated fat: 18g, Unsaturated fat: 6g

Difficulty rating: ★★☆☆

Tips for ingredient variations: Add slices of cooked sausage or ground beef for an extra protein boost.

Meat Lover's Breakfast Skillet (Bacon, Sausage, Eggs)

Number of servings: 4

Preparation time: 10 minutes

Cooking time: 20 minutes

Nutritional value per serving: Calories: 350, Carbs: 2g, Fiber: 0g, Sugars: 1g, Protein: 25g, Saturated fat: 20g, Unsaturated fat: 8g

Difficulty rating: ★★☆☆

Tips for ingredient variations: Add diced ham or ground beef for additional meat variety.

Directions:

1. Cook the diced bacon in a big skillet over medium heat until it's crispy. Remove and set aside.

2. In the same skillet, cook the sliced sausage until browned. Remove and set aside with the bacon.

3. Melt the butter in the skillet over medium heat.

4. Once the eggs are cracked into the skillet, scramble them until the desired doneness is achieved.

5. Return the bacon and sausage to the skillet, mixing with the eggs.

6. If using, sprinkle the shredded cheese over the mixture and cook until melted.

7. Serve warm, seasoned with sea salt and black pepper.

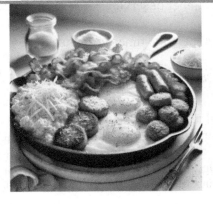

Ingredients:

• 4 slices bacon, chopped
• 4 sausage links, sliced
• 8 large eggs
• 1 cup shredded cheese (optional)
• Sea salt and black pepper to taste
• 2 tablespoons butter

Bone Broth Breakfast Soup

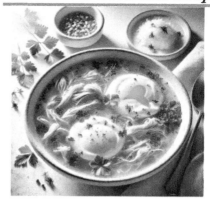

Ingredients:
- 4 cups bone broth
- 4 large eggs
- 1 cup cooked shredded chicken
- 1 tablespoon butter
- Sea salt and black pepper to taste
- Fresh herbs (optional)

Directions:
1. In a large pot, heat the bone broth over medium-high heat until it begins to simmer.
2. Add the shredded chicken to the pot and cook until heated through.
3. Crack the eggs directly into the simmering broth, one at a time, and poach for 3-4 minutes, or until the whites are set but the yolks remain runny.
4. Stir in the butter until melted.
5. Season with sea salt and black pepper to taste.
6. If preferred, top the soup with freshly chopped herbs after ladling it into dishes.

Number of servings: 4

Preparation time: 10 minutes

Cooking time: 20 minutes

Nutritional value per serving: Calories: 200, Carbs: 0g, Fiber: 0g, Sugars: 0g, Protein: 18g, Saturated fat: 6g, Unsaturated fat: 4g

Difficulty rating: ★★☆☆

Tips for ingredient variations: Add a splash of heavy cream for a richer broth or include cooked bacon bits for extra flavor.

Smoked Salmon and Scrambled Eggs

Number of servings: 2

Preparation time: 10 minutes

Cooking time: 10 minutes

Nutritional value per serving: Calories: 200, Carbs: 1g, Fiber: 0g, Sugars: 0g, Protein: 15g, Saturated fat: 10g, Unsaturated fat: 5g

Difficulty rating: ★★☆☆

Tips for ingredient variations: Add a squeeze of lemon juice over the eggs before serving for a fresh, tangy flavor.

Directions:
1. In a bowl, whisk together the eggs, heavy cream, sea salt, and black pepper until well combined.
2. Melt the butter in a non-stick skillet over medium heat.
3. Pour the egg mixture into the skillet and let it sit without stirring for about 30 seconds.
4. Using a spatula, gently whisk the eggs while cooking them until they softly scramble.
5. Just before the eggs are fully set, add the chopped smoked salmon and stir to combine.
6. Remove the skillet from the heat and garnish with fresh dill.
7. Serve immediately.

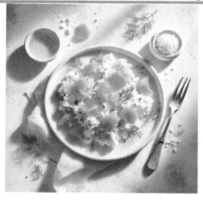

Ingredients:
- 4 large eggs
- 2 ounces smoked salmon, chopped
- 2 tablespoons heavy cream
- 1 tablespoon butter
- Sea salt and black pepper to taste
- Fresh dill, chopped, for garnish

Chicken Liver and Eggs

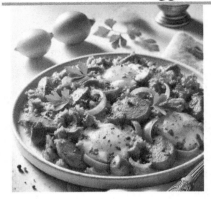

Ingredients:
• 4 large eggs
• 6 ounces chicken livers, cleaned and chopped
• 1 tablespoon butter
• 1 small onion, finely chopped
• Sea salt and black pepper to taste
• 1 tablespoon fresh parsley, chopped (optional)

Directions:
1. In a bowl, whisk the eggs with sea salt and black pepper until well combined.
2. Melt the butter in a skillet over medium-high heat.
3. Add the chopped onion to the skillet and cook for 3-4 minutes, or until it turns translucent.
4. Add the chicken livers to the skillet and cook, stirring occasionally, until they are browned and cooked through, about 5-6 minutes.
5. Reduce the heat to medium and pour the beaten eggs over the chicken livers and onions.
6. Stir gently until the eggs are fully cooked and scrambled.
7. Garnish with fresh parsley if desired.
8. Serve immediately.

Number of servings: 2

Preparation time: 10 minutes

Cooking time: 15 minutes

Nutritional value per serving: Calories: 250, Carbs: 2g, Fiber: 0g, Sugars: 1g, Protein: 20g, Saturated fat: 8g, Unsaturated fat: 7g

Difficulty rating: ★★★☆☆

Tips for ingredient variations: Add a splash of heavy cream to the eggs before whisking for a creamier texture.

Lamb Kidney and Egg Scramble

Number of servings: 2

Preparation time: 15 minutes

Cooking time: 15 minutes

Nutritional value per serving: Calories: 230, Carbs: 2g, Fiber: 0g, Sugars: 1g, Protein: 22g, Saturated fat: 7g, Unsaturated fat: 8g

Difficulty rating: ★★★☆☆

Tips for ingredient variations: Add a small handful of chopped spinach to the eggs before scrambling for added nutrients and color.

Directions:
1. In a bowl, whisk the eggs with sea salt and black pepper until well combined.
2. Melt the butter in a skillet over medium-high heat.
3. Add the chopped shallot to the skillet and sauté until it becomes translucent, about 2-3 minutes.
4. Add the chopped lamb kidneys to the skillet and cook, stirring occasionally, until they are browned and cooked through, about 5-6 minutes.
5. Reduce the heat to medium and pour the beaten eggs over the lamb kidneys and shallots.
6. Stir gently until the eggs are fully cooked and scrambled.
7. Garnish with fresh thyme if desired.
8. Serve immediately.

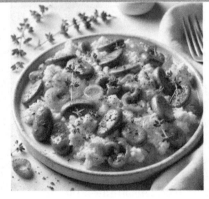

Ingredients:
• 4 large eggs
• 2 lamb kidneys, cleaned and chopped
• 1 tablespoon butter
• 1 small shallot, finely chopped
• Sea salt and black pepper to taste
• 1 teaspoon fresh thyme, chopped (optional)

Duck Egg Omelet

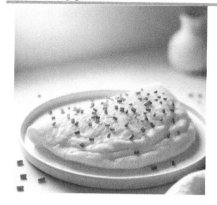

Ingredients:
- 4 duck eggs
- 2 tablespoons heavy cream
- 2 tablespoons butter
- 1 tablespoon fresh chives, chopped
- Sea salt and black pepper to taste

Directions:

1. In a medium bowl, whisk together the duck eggs, heavy cream, sea salt, and black pepper until well combined.

2. Heat the butter in a non-stick skillet over medium heat until melted and slightly bubbly.

3. Pour the egg mixture into the skillet and cook undisturbed for about 2-3 minutes, or until the edges start to set.

4. Sprinkle the chopped chives evenly over the omelet.

5. Using a spatula, carefully fold the omelet in half and continue to cook for another 2-3 minutes, until the eggs are fully set.

6. Transfer the omelet to a platter and enjoy it hot.

Number of servings: 2

Preparation time: 5 minutes

Cooking time: 10 minutes

Nutritional value per serving: Calories: 220, Carbs: 1g, Fiber: 0g, Sugars: 0g, Protein: 14g, Saturated fat: 16g, Unsaturated fat: 6g

Difficulty rating: ★★☆☆

Tips for ingredient variations: Add 2 tablespoons of crumbled goat cheese for extra richness and flavor.

Beef Liver and Onion Omelet

Number of servings: 2

Preparation time: 10 minutes

Cooking time: 15 minutes

Nutritional value per serving: Calories: 280, Carbs: 3g, Fiber: 0g, Sugars: 1g, Protein: 22g, Saturated fat: 14g, Unsaturated fat: 8g

Difficulty rating: ★★★☆☆

Tips for ingredient variations: Add ¼ cup of shredded cheddar cheese to the egg mixture for a cheesy twist.

Directions:

1. In a medium bowl, whisk together the eggs, heavy cream, sea salt, and black pepper until well combined.

2. In a skillet over medium heat, melt one tablespoon of butter. Add the thinly sliced onions and sauté until soft and caramelized, about 5 minutes.

3. Add the chopped beef liver to the skillet and cook for another 2 minutes, until heated through. Remove the liver and onions from the skillet and set aside.

4. Add the remaining tablespoon of butter to the skillet and let it melt.

5. Pour the egg mixture into the skillet and cook undisturbed for about 2-3 minutes, until the edges start to set.

6. Spread the liver and onion mixture evenly over one half of the omelet.

7. Using a spatula, carefully fold the omelet in half over the filling and continue to cook for another 2-3 minutes, until the eggs are fully set.

8. Transfer the omelet to a platter and serve it warm.

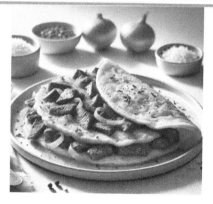

Ingredients:
- 4 large eggs
- ½ cup cooked beef liver, chopped
- ½ small onion, thinly sliced
- 2 tablespoons heavy cream
- 2 tablespoons butter
- Sea salt and black pepper to taste

Cream Cheese and Egg Puffs

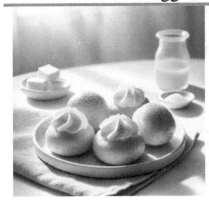

Ingredients:
- 6 large eggs
- 4 ounces cream cheese, softened
- 1 tablspoon butter, melted
- Sea salt and black pepper to taste

Directions:

1. Preheat your oven to 375° F (190° C). Use butter or cooking spray to grease a muffin pan.
2. In a medium bowl, beat the eggs until smooth and well combined.
3. Add the softened cream cheese to the eggs and mix until smooth. Season with sea salt and black pepper.
4. Evenly fill each cup of the muffin tin with the mixture, filling it to about three-quarters of the way.
5. Melt the butter and drizzle it over the top of each puff.
6. Bake for 20 minutes, or until the puffs are set and golden brown.
7. Take out the muffin tray from the oven, and then let the puffs a few minutes to cool before taking them out of the tin.
8. Serve warm or at room temperature.

Number of servings: 4

Preparation time: 10 minutes

Cooking time: 20 minutes

Nutritional value per serving: Calories: 150, Carbs: 2g, Fiber: 0g, Sugars: 1g, Protein: 8g, Saturated fat: 10g, Unsaturated fat: 4g

Difficulty rating:
★★☆☆☆

Tips for ingredient variations: Add 1 tablespoon of fresh herbs like chives or parsley to the egg mixture for a burst of flavor.

Starters

Bacon-Wrapped Scallops

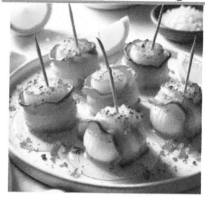

Ingredients:

- 12 large sea scallops
- 12 slices bacon
- 2 tablespoons butter, melted
- Sea salt and black pepper to taste
- Lemon wedges for serving

Directions:

1. Preheat your oven to 400° F (200° C).
2. Place a piece of bacon around each scallop and fasten it with a toothpick.
3. Place the bacon-wrapped scallops on a baking sheet.
4. Brush the scallops with melted butter and season with sea salt and black pepper.
5. Bake for 15 to 20 minutes, or until the scallops are cooked through and the bacon is crispy.
6. Serve immediately with lemon wedges.

Number of servings: 4

Preparation time: 15 minutes

Cooking time: 20 minutes

Nutritional value per serving: Calories: 300, Carbs: 0g, Fiber: 0g, Sugars: 0g, Protein: 25g, Saturated fat: 12g, Unsaturated fat: 8g

Difficulty rating: ★★☆☆

Tips for ingredient variations: Add a sprinkle of smoked paprika or garlic powder to the butter for extra flavor.

Beef Tartare

Number of servings: 4

Preparation time: 20 minutes

Cooking time: None

Nutritional value per serving: Calories: 250, Carbs: 1g, Fiber: 0g, Sugars: 0g, Protein: 28g, Saturated fat: 6g, Unsaturated fat: 8g

Difficulty rating: ★★★☆☆

Tips for ingredient variations: Add a dash of hot sauce or finely chopped pickles for extra zing.

Directions:

1. In a large bowl, combine the chopped beef, capers, shallots, Dijon mustard, Worcestershire sauce, sea salt, and black pepper. Mix well.
2. Divide the beef mixture into four portions and shape each into a patty.
3. Make a small indentation in the center of each patty and place an egg yolk in each indentation.
4. Sprinkle with chopped fresh parsley and serve immediately.

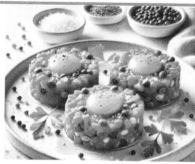

Ingredients:

- 1 lb beef tenderloin, finely chopped
- 1 egg yolk
- 2 tablespoons capers, drained and chopped
- 2 tablespoons finely chopped shallots
- 1 tablespoon Dijon mustard
- 1 tablespoon Worcestershire sauce
- Sea salt and black pepper to taste
- 1 tablespoon chopped fresh parsley

Chicken Liver Pâté

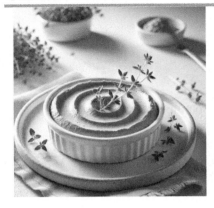

Ingredients:
- 1 lb chicken livers, cleaned and trimmed
- 1 small onion, finely chopped
- 2 cloves garlic, minced
- 1/2 cup butter, divided
- 2 tablespoons heavy cream
- Sea salt and black pepper to taste
- 1 tablespoon fresh thyme leaves

Directions:

1. Melt two tablespoons of butter in a large skillet over medium heat. Add the onion and garlic, cooking until softened.

2. After adding the chicken livers to the skillet, cook them for five to seven minutes, or until the middle is no longer pink.

3. Pour the mixture into a food processor. Add the remaining butter, heavy cream, sea salt, black pepper, and thyme leaves. Blend until smooth.

4. Before serving, spoon the pâté into a serving dish and place it in the refrigerator for at least an hour.

Number of servings: 8

Preparation time: 15 minutes

Cooking time: 20 minutes

Nutritional value per serving: Calories: 180, Carbs: 1g, Fiber: 0g, Sugars: 0g, Protein: 14g, Saturated fat: 10g, Unsaturated fat: 4g

Difficulty rating: ★★★☆☆

Tips for ingredient variations: Add a splash of brandy or cognac during cooking for a richer flavor.

Deviled Eggs with Bacon Bits

Number of servings: 6

Preparation time: 15 minutes

Cooking time: 10 minutes

Nutritional value per serving: Calories: 120, Carbs: 1g, Fiber: 0g, Sugars: 0g, Protein: 7g, Saturated fat: 3g, Unsaturated fat: 4g

Difficulty rating: ★★☆☆☆

Tips for ingredient variations: Add a dash of hot sauce or a sprinkle of smoked paprika for extra flavor.

Directions:

1. Place the eggs in a saucepan and cover with water. Bring to a boil, then reduce heat and simmer for 10 minutes. Drain and cool in an ice bath.

2. Peel the eggs and cut them in half lengthwise. Remove the yolks and place them in a bowl.

3. Mash the yolks with a fork and stir in the mayonnaise, Dijon mustard, paprika, sea salt, and black pepper until smooth.

4. The yolk mixture can be piped or spooned back into the egg whites.

5. Top with crumbled bacon and chopped chives. Serve immediately.

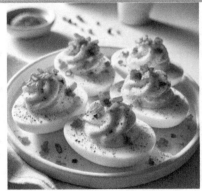

Ingredients:
- 6 large eggs
- 3 tablespoons mayonnaise
- 1 teaspoon Dijon mustard
- 1/4 teaspoon paprika
- Sea salt and black pepper to taste
- 2 slices bacon, cooked and crumbled
- Chopped chives for garnish

Pork Rind Nachos

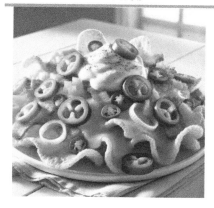

Ingredients:
- 4 cups pork rinds
- 1 cup shredded cheddar cheese
- 1/2 cup sour cream
- 1/4 cup sliced jalapeños
- 1/4 cup diced onions
- 1/4 cup diced tomatoes
- Sea salt and black pepper to taste

Directions:
1. Preheat your oven to 350° F (175° C).
2. Spread the pork rinds evenly on a baking sheet.
3. Sprinkle the shredded cheddar cheese over the pork rinds.
4. Bake in the preheated oven for 5 minutes, or until the cheese is melted and bubbly.
5. Remove from the oven and top with sour cream, sliced jalapeños, diced onions, and diced tomatoes.
6. Season with sea salt and black pepper to taste. Serve immediately.

Number of servings: 4

Preparation time: 10 minutes

Cooking time: 5 minutes

Nutritional value per serving: Calories: 320, Carbs: 2g, Fiber: 0g, Sugars: 1g, Protein: 24g, Saturated fat: 12g, Unsaturated fat: 8g

Difficulty rating: ★★☆☆

Tips for ingredient variations: Add cooked ground beef or shredded chicken for extra protein and flavor.

Cheese-Stuffed Mushrooms (Carnivore Version)

Number of servings: 4

Preparation time: 15 minutes

Cooking time: 20 minutes

Nutritional value per serving: Calories: 220, Carbs: 3g, Fiber: 1g, Sugars: 2g, Protein: 10g, Saturated fat: 14g, Unsaturated fat: 6g

Difficulty rating: ★★☆☆

Tips for ingredient variations: Add 2 tablespoons of cooked and crumbled bacon to the cheese mixture for extra flavor.

Directions:
1. Preheat your oven to 375° F (190° C).
2. Take off the stems and clean the mushrooms. Place the caps of the mushrooms aside.
3. In a medium bowl, mix together the cream cheese, Parmesan cheese, mozzarella cheese, chives, garlic powder, sea salt, and black pepper until well combined.
4. Stuff each mushroom cap with the cheese mixture.
5. Place the stuffed mushrooms on a baking sheet and bake for 20 minutes, or until the mushrooms are tender and the cheese is golden brown.
6. Serve warm.

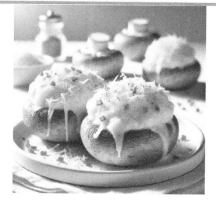

Ingredients:
- 12 large white mushrooms, stems removed
- 8 ounces cream cheese, softened
- 1/2 cup grated Parmesan cheese
- 1/2 cup shredded mozzarella cheese
- 2 tablespoons chopped fresh chives
- 1 teaspoon garlic powder
- Sea salt and black pepper to taste

Beef Carpaccio

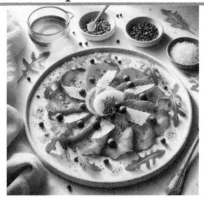

Directions:
1. Arrange the thinly sliced beef tenderloin on a large serving platter.
2. Pour the lemon juice and olive oil onto the steak.
3. Sprinkle with capers, shaved Parmesan cheese, sea salt, and black pepper.
4. Garnish with fresh arugula if desired.
5. Serve immediately.

Number of servings: 4

Preparation time: 10 minutes

Cooking time: 0 minutes

Nutritional value per serving:
Calories: 250, Carbs: 1g, Fiber: 0g, Sugars: 0g, Protein: 22g, Saturated fat: 6g, Unsaturated fat: 12g

Difficulty rating: ★★☆☆

Tips for ingredient variations:
Add thin slices of radish or drizzle with a balsamic reduction for additional flavor.

Ingredients:
• 1 pound beef tenderloin, very thinly sliced
• 3 tablespoons extra-virgin olive oil
• 2 tablespoons capers, drained
• 1/4 cup shaved Parmesan cheese
• 1 tablespoon lemon juice
• Sea salt and black pepper to taste
• Fresh arugula (optional)

Bone Marrow Butter on Toasted Carnivore Bread

Number of servings: 4

Preparation time: 10 minutes

Cooking time: 15 minutes

Nutritional value per serving:
Calories: 380, Carbs: 1g, Fiber: 0g, Sugars: 0g, Protein: 7g, Saturated fat: 30g, Unsaturated fat: 10g

Difficulty rating: ★★★☆☆

Tips for ingredient variations:
Add a touch of garlic powder or smoked paprika to the bone marrow butter for an extra burst of flavor.

Directions:
1. Preheat your oven to 450° F (230° C).
2. Place the marrow bones on a baking sheet and roast for 15 minutes, or until the marrow is soft and bubbling.
3. Scoop the marrow into a bowl and mix with the softened butter, chopped parsley, sea salt, and black pepper.
4. Toast the carnivore bread slices until golden brown.
5. Spread the bone marrow butter on the toasted bread and serve warm.

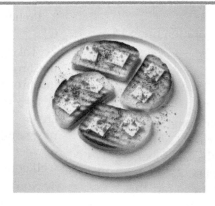

Ingredients:
• 4 beef marrow bones
• 1/2 cup unsalted butter, softened
• 1 tablespoon chopped fresh parsley
• Sea salt and black pepper to taste
• 8 slices of carnivore bread (recipe available separately)

Prosciutto-Wrapped Asparagus

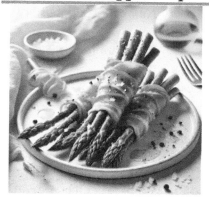

Ingredients:
- 1 bunch asparagus spears, trimmed
- 12 slices prosciutto
- 1 tablespoon olive oil
- Sea salt and black pepper to taste

Directions:

1. Preheat your oven to 400° F (200° C).
2. Wrap each asparagus spear with a slice of prosciutto.
3. Arrange the wrapped asparagus on a baking sheet.
4. Drizzle with olive oil and season with sea salt and black pepper.
5. Bake for 15 minutes, or until the asparagus is tender and the prosciutto is crispy.
6. Serve warm.

Number of servings: 4

Preparation time: 10 minutes

Cooking time: 15 minutes

Nutritional value per serving: Calories: 150, Carbs: 2g, Fiber: 1g, Sugars: 1g, Protein: 10g, Saturated fat: 4g, Unsaturated fat: 8g

Difficulty rating: ★★☆☆☆

Tips for ingredient variations: Sprinkle with grated Parmesan cheese before baking for an added layer of flavor.

Crispy Chicken Skins

Number of servings: 4

Preparation time: 10 minutes

Cooking time: 45 minutes

Nutritional value per serving: Calories: 200, Carbs: 0g, Fiber: 0g, Sugars: 0g, Protein: 15g, Saturated fat: 4g, Unsaturated fat: 10g

Difficulty rating: ★★☆☆☆

Tips for ingredient variations: Sprinkle with smoked paprika or garlic powder before baking for added flavor.

Directions:

1. Preheat your oven to 375° F (190° C).
2. Pat the chicken skins dry with paper towels.
3. Season the skins with sea salt and black pepper after brushing them with olive oil on both sides.
4. Place the skins on a baking sheet lined with parchment paper.
5. Bake for 45 minutes, or until the skins are crispy and golden brown.
6. Before serving, allow the skins to cool slightly.

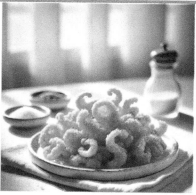

Ingredients:
- Skins from 4 chicken breasts
- 1 tablespoon olive oil
- Sea salt and black pepper to taste

Lamb Meatballs with Mint Sauce

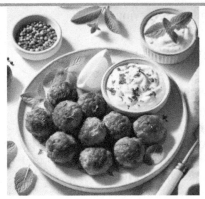

Ingredients:

- 1 lb ground lamb
- 1 egg
- 1/4 cup grated Parmesan cheese
- 2 cloves garlic, minced
- 1 tablespoon fresh mint, chopped
- 1 tablespoon fresh parsley, chopped
- Sea salt and black pepper to taste

Mint Sauce:

- 1/2 cup Greek yogurt (optional for strict carnivore: replace with blended lamb fat)
- 1 tablespoon fresh mint, chopped
- 1 tablespoon lemon juice
- Sea salt to taste

Directions:

1. Preheat your oven to 375° F (190° C).

2. In a large bowl, combine the ground lamb, egg, Parmesan cheese, minced garlic, mint, parsley, salt, and pepper. Mix until well combined.

3. Form the mixture into meatballs, about 1 inch in diameter, and place them on a baking sheet.

4. The meatballs should be baked for 20 to 25 minutes, or until they are thoroughly cooked and have a browned exterior.

5. While the meatballs are baking, prepare the mint sauce by combining the Greek yogurt (or blended lamb fat), chopped mint, lemon juice, and salt in a small bowl. Mix well.

6. Serve the meatballs warm with the mint sauce on the side.

Number of servings: 4

Preparation time: 20 minutes

Cooking time: 25 minutes

Nutritional value per serving: Calories: 350, Carbs: 2g, Fiber: 0g, Sugars: 1g, Protein: 22g, Saturated fat: 15g, Unsaturated fat: 12g

Difficulty rating:
★★☆☆

Tips for ingredient variations: For a richer flavor, add 1 teaspoon of cumin to the meatball mixture.

Shrimp Cocktail (with Carnivore Sauce)

Number of servings: 4

Preparation time: 10 minutes

Cooking time: 5 minutes

Nutritional value per serving: Calories: 250, Carbs: 1g, Fiber: 0g, Sugars: 0g, Protein: 20g, Saturated fat: 5g, Unsaturated fat: 15g

Difficulty rating:
★☆☆☆

Tips for ingredient variations: For extra zest, add 1 teaspoon of hot sauce to the carnivore sauce.

Directions:

1. Bring a large pot of water to a boil and squeeze in the juice of half a lemon. Add a pinch of sea salt.

2. Add the shrimp to the boiling water and cook for 2-3 minutes, or until they turn pink and are cooked through.

3. Drain the shrimp and transfer them to a bowl of ice water to cool.

4. In a small bowl, whisk together the mayonnaise, horseradish, lemon juice, Worcestershire sauce (if using), and salt to make the carnivore sauce.

5. Serve the chilled shrimp with the carnivore sauce on the side.

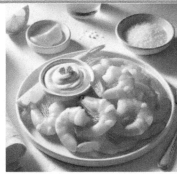

Ingredients:

- 1 lb large shrimp, peeled and deveined
- 1 lemon, halved
- Sea salt to taste

Carnivore Sauce:

- 1/2 cup mayonnaise
- 2 tablespoons prepared horseradish
- 1 tablespoon lemon juice
- 1 teaspoon Worcestershire sauce (optional)
- Sea salt to taste

Carnivore Charcuterie Board

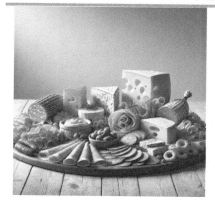

Ingredients:

- 8 ounces sliced prosciutto
- 8 ounces sliced salami
- 8 ounces sliced chorizo
- 8 ounces smoked sausage, sliced
- 8 ounces cheese (e.g., cheddar, gouda, blue cheese)
- 4 ounces pate (optional)
- 4 ounces pork rinds
- 4 ounces olives (optional)
- 2 ounces pickles (optional)

Directions:

1. On a large serving board, arrange the sliced prosciutto, salami, chorizo, and smoked sausage.
2. Add the slices of cheese around the meats.
3. Place the pate, if using, in a small dish and add it to the board.
4. Fill in the remaining spaces with pork rinds, olives, and pickles (if using).
5. Serve immediately and enjoy with your favorite carnivore-friendly beverages.

Number of servings: 6

Preparation time: 15 minutes

Nutritional value per serving: Calories: 450, Carbs: 2g, Fiber: 0g, Sugars: 1g, Protein: 28g, Saturated fat: 22g, Unsaturated fat: 18g

Difficulty rating: ★☆☆☆☆

Tips for ingredient variations: Add some beef jerky or smoked fish to diversify the protein options.

Grilled Octopus Tentacles

Number of servings: 4

Preparation time: 15 minutes

Cooking time: 1 hour 15 minutes

Nutritional value per serving: Calories: 250, Carbs: 1g, Fiber: 0g, Sugars: 0g, Protein: 35g, Saturated fat: 2g, Unsaturated fat: 10g

Difficulty rating: ★★★☆☆

Tips for ingredient variations: Add a dash of chili flakes to the olive oil mixture for a spicy kick.

Directions:

1. In a big pot, bring the water to a boil. Add the lemon halves and a pinch of sea salt.
2. Submerge the octopus tentacles in the boiling water and cook for 1 hour, or until tender.
3. Remove the tentacles from the water and let them cool slightly.
4. Preheat your grill to medium-high heat.
5. In a small bowl, mix together the olive oil, minced garlic, sea salt, black pepper, and paprika.
6. Brush the tentacles with the olive oil mixture.
7. Grill the tentacles for 3-4 minutes on each side, until they are charred and crispy.
8. Serve warm with additional lemon wedges.

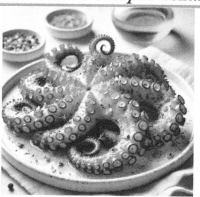

Ingredients:

- 2 lbs octopus tentacles
- 1 lemon, halved
- 2 cloves garlic, minced
- 2 tablespoons olive oil
- Sea salt and black pepper to taste
- 1 teaspoon paprika

Duck Liver Mousse

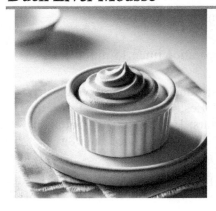

Ingredients:
- 1 lb duck liver, cleaned and trimmed
- 1/2 cup heavy cream
- 1/4 cup butter, softened
- 1 small shallot, minced
- 2 cloves garlic, minced
- 1 tablespoon brandy (optional)
- Sea salt and black pepper to taste

Directions:

1. In a medium skillet, melt 2 tablespoons of butter over medium heat. Sauté the minced shallot and garlic until they become tender.

2. Add the duck liver to the skillet and cook for 3-4 minutes on each side, until browned and cooked through.

3. Transfer the cooked liver, shallot, and garlic to a food processor. Stir in the heavy cream, brandy (if using), and the remaining butter. Season with sea salt and black pepper.

4. Blend until smooth and creamy.

5. Spoon the mousse into ramekins or a serving dish, and refrigerate for at least 1 hour before serving.

6. Serve chilled with pork rinds or on its own.

Number of servings: 6

Preparation time: 20 minutes

Cooking time: 10 minutes

Nutritional value per serving:
Calories: 320, Carbs: 2g, Fiber: 0g, Sugars: 1g, Protein: 16g, Saturated fat: 20g, Unsaturated fat: 10g

Difficulty rating: ★★★☆☆

Tips for ingredient variations: For a richer flavor, add a pinch of nutmeg or allspice to the mousse mixture.

Carnivore Sushi (Beef and Tuna)

Number of servings: 4

Preparation time: 20 minutes

Cooking time: 0 minutes

Nutritional value per serving:
Calories: 200, Carbs: 0g, Fiber: 0g, Sugars: 0g, Protein: 30g, Saturated fat: 3g, Unsaturated fat: 7g

Difficulty rating: ★☆☆☆

Tips for ingredient variations:
Add a thin slice of avocado inside the rolls for a creamy texture.

Directions:

1. Lay out the slices of beef and tuna on a clean surface.

2. Roll the beef slices tightly into sushi rolls.

3. Roll the tuna slices tightly into sushi rolls.

4. Arrange the beef and tuna rolls on a serving plate.

5. If preferred, serve with wasabi and soy sauce on the side for dipping.

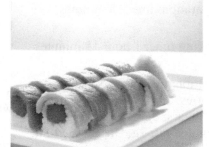

Ingredients:
- 8 ounces beef tenderloin, thinly sliced
- 8 ounces sushi-grade tuna, thinly sliced
- 2 tablespoons soy sauce (optional, for dipping)
- 1 teaspoon wasabi paste (optional, for dipping)

Bacon-Wrapped Jalapeño Poppers

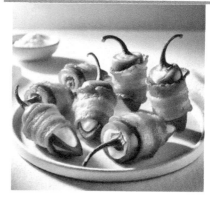

Ingredients:
• 12 jalapeño peppers, halved and seeded
• 8 ounces cream cheese, softened
• 12 slices bacon, cut in half

Directions:
1. Preheat your oven to 400° F (200° C).
2. Spoon cream cheese into each half of a jalapeño.
3. Put a half slice of bacon around each filled jalapeño half and, if needed, secure with a toothpick.
4. Place the bacon-wrapped jalapeños on a baking sheet lined with parchment paper.
5. Bake for 20-25 minutes, or until the bacon is crispy and the jalapeños are tender.
6. Allow to cool for a few minutes before serving warm.

Number of servings: 6

Preparation time: 15 minutes

Cooking time: 25 minutes

Nutritional value per serving:
Calories: 150, Carbs: 2g, Fiber: 0g, Sugars: 1g, Protein: 5g, Saturated fat: 9g, Unsaturated fat: 3g

Difficulty rating: ★★☆☆☆

Tips for ingredient variations: Add shredded cheddar cheese to the cream cheese for extra flavor.

Salmon Caviar on Egg Slices

Number of servings: 4

Preparation time: 10 minutes

Cooking time: 10 minutes

Nutritional value per serving:
Calories: 90, Carbs: 1g, Fiber: 0g, Sugars: 0g, Protein: 8g, Saturated fat: 2g, Unsaturated fat: 3g

Difficulty rating: ★☆☆☆☆

Tips for ingredient variations: Add a small dollop of crème fraîche under the caviar for added richness.

Directions:
1. Put the eggs in a pot and pour cold water over them.
2. After bringing to a boil, lower heat, and simmer for nine minutes.
3. Remove the eggs from the hot water and cool under cold running water.
4. Peel the eggs and slice each egg into four rounds.
5. Place a small dollop of salmon caviar on top of each egg slice.
6. Garnish with fresh dill and serve immediately.

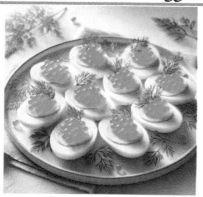

Ingredients:
• 4 large eggs
• 4 tablespoons salmon caviar
• Fresh dill, for garnish

Main Dishes

Ribeye Steak with Garlic Butter

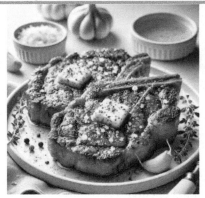

Ingredients:
• 2 ribeye steaks, about 12 oz each
• 2 tablespoons olive oil
• Sea salt and cracked black pepper to taste
• 4 tablespoons unsalted butter
• 4 cloves garlic, minced
• 1 tablespoon fresh thyme, chopped

Directions:
1. Preheat your grill to high heat.
2. Rub the ribeye steaks with olive oil and season generously with sea salt and cracked black pepper on both sides.
3. For medium-rare, grill the steaks for 4-5 minutes on each side, or until done to your preference.
4. While the steaks are grilling, melt the butter in a small saucepan over medium heat. Add the minced garlic and cook for 1-2 minutes until fragrant. Stir in the chopped thyme.
5. After taking the steaks from the grill, rest them for five minutes.
6. Drizzle the garlic butter over the steaks before serving.

Number of servings: 2

Preparation time: 10 minutes

Cooking time: 15 minutes

Nutritional value per serving: Calories: 650, Carbs: 1g, Fiber: 0g, Sugars: 0g, Protein: 45g, Saturated fat: 25g, Unsaturated fat: 22g

Difficulty rating: ★★☆☆

Tips for ingredient variations: Add a teaspoon of lemon juice to the garlic butter for a bright, tangy flavor.

Slow Cooker Beef Brisket

Number of servings: 6

Preparation time: 15 minutes

Cooking time: 8 hours

Nutritional value per serving: Calories: 420, Carbs: 2g, Fiber: 0g, Sugars: 0g, Protein: 45g, Saturated fat: 12g, Unsaturated fat: 18g

Difficulty rating: ★★☆☆

Tips for ingredient variations: Add a splash of Worcestershire sauce to the beef broth for added depth of flavor.

Directions:
1. In a small bowl, combine sea salt, cracked black pepper, smoked paprika, garlic powder, and onion powder.
2. Make sure the beef brisket is evenly coated with the spice mixture by rubbing it all over.
3. Place the brisket in the slow cooker and pour the beef broth around the sides.
4. For eight hours, or when the brisket is soft and easily shreds with a fork, cover and simmer on low.
5. Remove the brisket from the slow cooker and let it rest for 10 minutes before slicing against the grain.

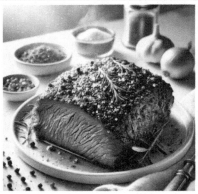

Ingredients:
• 1 (3 lb) beef brisket
• 2 tablespoons sea salt
• 1 tablespoon cracked black pepper
• 2 teaspoons smoked paprika
• 2 teaspoons garlic powder
• 1 teaspoon onion powder
• 1 cup beef broth

Grilled Lamb Chops

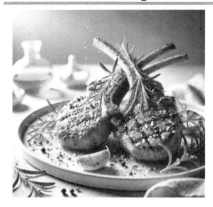

Ingredients:
- 8 lamb chops, about 1 inch thick
- 3 tablespoons olive oil
- 1 tablespoon fresh rosemary, chopped
- 2 cloves garlic, minced
- Sea salt and cracked black pepper to taste

Directions:
1. Preheat your grill to medium-high heat.
2. In a small bowl, mix the olive oil, chopped rosemary, minced garlic, sea salt, and cracked black pepper.
3. Rub the olive oil mixture over the lamb chops, ensuring they are evenly coated.
4. Grill the lamb chops for about 5-6 minutes per side for medium-rare, or until they reach your desired level of doneness.
5. Remove the lamb chops from the grill and let them rest for 5 minutes before serving.

Number of servings: 4

Preparation time: 10 minutes

Cooking time: 15 minutes

Nutritional value per serving: Calories: 360, Carbs: 0g, Fiber: 0g, Sugars: 0g, Protein: 25g, Saturated fat: 12g, Unsaturated fat: 18g

Difficulty rating: ★★☆☆

Tips for ingredient variations: Add a squeeze of lemon juice over the lamb chops before serving for a fresh, tangy finish.

Beef Tenderloin with Blue Cheese Crust

Number of servings: 4

Preparation time: 15 minutes

Cooking time: 45 minutes

Nutritional value per serving: Calories: 510, Carbs: 2g, Fiber: 0g, Sugars: 0g, Protein: 45g, Saturated fat: 22g, Unsaturated fat: 20g

Difficulty rating: ★★★☆☆

Tips for ingredient variations: Substitute the blue cheese with gorgonzola for a slightly milder flavor.

Directions:
1. Preheat your oven to 400°F (200°C).
2. Rub the beef tenderloin with olive oil and season generously with sea salt and cracked black pepper.
3. In a small bowl, mix the crumbled blue cheese, softened butter, and chopped parsley.
4. Sear the tenderloin in a hot skillet over medium-high heat for about 2-3 minutes per side, until browned.
5. Transfer the tenderloin to a baking dish and spread the blue cheese mixture over the top.
6. Bake for 35-40 minutes, or until the tenderloin reaches an internal temperature of 135°F (57°C) for medium-rare.
7. Remove from the oven and let it rest for 10 minutes before slicing.

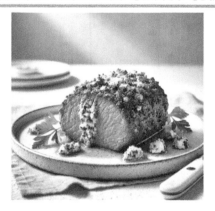

Ingredients:
- 1 (2 lb) beef tenderloin
- 2 tablespoons olive oil
- Sea salt and cracked black pepper to taste
- 4 ounces blue cheese, crumbled
- 2 tablespoons butter, softened
- 1 tablespoon fresh parsley, chopped

Smoked Beef Ribs

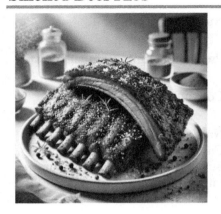

Ingredients:
• 4 beef short ribs
• 2 tablespoons coarse sea salt
• 1 tablespoon cracked black pepper
• 2 teaspoons garlic powder
• 1 teaspoon onion powder
• 1 teaspoon smoked paprika

Directions:
1. Preheat your smoker to 225°F (107°C).
2. In a small bowl, combine sea salt, cracked black pepper, garlic powder, onion powder, and smoked paprika.
3. Rub the spice mixture all over the beef short ribs, ensuring they are evenly coated.
4. Place the ribs in the smoker and cook for about 6 hours, or until they reach an internal temperature of 205°F (96°C) and are tender.
5. Before serving, take the ribs out of the smoker and rest for 10 minutes.

Number of servings: 4

Preparation time: 15 minutes

Cooking time: 6 hours

Nutritional value per serving:
Calories: 620, Carbs: 1g, Fiber: 0g, Sugars: 0g, Protein: 45g, Saturated fat: 20g, Unsaturated fat: 25g

Difficulty rating: ★★★☆☆

Tips for ingredient variations:
Brush the ribs with a low-carb BBQ sauce during the last hour of smoking for added flavor.

Ground Beef Carnivore Chili

Number of servings: 6

Preparation time: 10 minutes

Cooking time: 1 hour

Nutritional value per serving:
Calories: 320, Carbs: 2g, Fiber: 1g, Sugars: 0g, Protein: 25g, Saturated fat: 8g, Unsaturated fat: 15g

Difficulty rating: ★☆☆☆☆

Tips for ingredient variations: For a richer flavor, add 1 tablespoon of cocoa powder to the chili.

Directions:
1. In a large pot, cook the ground beef over medium heat until browned, breaking it up with a spoon as it cooks.
2. Drain any excess fat and return the beef to the pot.
3. Add the beef bone broth, smoked paprika, chili powder, garlic powder, onion powder, sea salt, and black pepper. Stir well to combine.
4. Bring the mixture to a boil, then reduce the heat to low and simmer for 45 minutes to 1 hour, stirring occasionally, until the chili thickens to your desired consistency.
5. Serve hot.

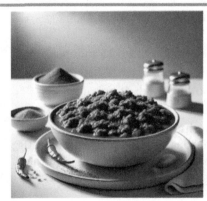

Ingredients:
• 2 lbs ground beef
• 1 cup beef bone broth
• 1 tablespoon smoked paprika
• 1 tablespoon chili powder
• 1 teaspoon garlic powder
• 1 teaspoon onion powder
• 1 teaspoon sea salt
• ½ teaspoon black pepper

Beef and Lamb Meatloaf

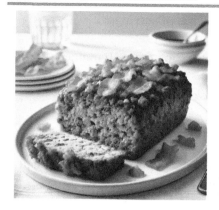

Ingredients:

- 1 lb ground beef
- 1 lb ground lamb
- 1 large egg
- ½ cup grated Parmesan cheese
- 1 teaspoon garlic powder
- 1 teaspoon onion powder
- 1 teaspoon dried thyme
- 1 teaspoon sea salt
- ½ teaspoon black pepper
- 4 slices bacon, chopped

Directions:

1. Preheat your oven to 350°F (175°C).
2. In a large bowl, combine the ground beef, ground lamb, egg, grated Parmesan cheese, garlic powder, onion powder, dried thyme, sea salt, and black pepper. Mix until well combined.
3. Shape the mixture into a loaf and place it in a loaf pan.
4. Over the meatloaf, scatter the diced bacon.
5. Bake the meatloaf for one hour, or until it is cooked through and the internal temperature reaches 70°C, or 160°F.
6. Prior to slicing and serving, rest the meatloaf for ten minutes.

Number of servings: 6

Preparation time: 15 minutes

Cooking time: 1 hour

Nutritional value per serving:
Calories: 400, Carbs: 1g, Fiber: 0g, Sugars: 0g, Protein: 28g, Saturated fat: 16g, Unsaturated fat: 12g

Difficulty rating: ★★☆☆

Tips for ingredient variations: Add 1 tablespoon of Worcestershire sauce to the meat mixture for extra depth of flavor.

Braised Short Ribs

Number of servings: 4

Preparation time: 15 minutes

Cooking time: 3 hours

Nutritional value per serving:
Calories: 620, Carbs: 3g, Fiber: 0g, Sugars: 1g, Protein: 40g, Saturated fat: 22g, Unsaturated fat: 25g

Difficulty rating: ★★★☆☆

Tips for ingredient variations: Add 1 teaspoon of smoked paprika to the braising liquid for a smoky flavor.

Directions:

1. Preheat your oven to 325°F (165°C).
2. In a large Dutch oven, heat the olive oil over medium-high heat.
3. Season the short ribs with sea salt and black pepper, then brown them on all sides in the Dutch oven. Remove and set aside.
4. Add the minced garlic to the pot and sauté for 1 minute.
5. Scrape up any browned bits from the bottom of the saucepan as you stir in the tomato paste, beef bone broth, and red wine.
6. Return the short ribs to the pot and add the fresh thyme.
7. Cover and braise in the oven for 3 hours, or until the meat is tender and falling off the bone.
8. Remove the thyme sprigs before serving.

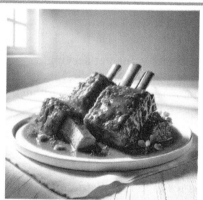

Ingredients:

- 4 lbs beef short ribs
- 2 tablespoons olive oil
- 1 cup beef bone broth
- 1 cup dry red wine
- 1 tablespoon tomato paste
- 2 cloves garlic, minced
- 1 teaspoon sea salt
- ½ teaspoon black pepper
- 2 sprigs fresh thyme

Grilled T-Bone Steak

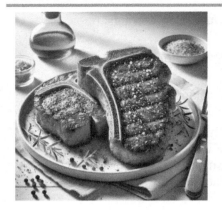

Ingredients:
- 2 (1 lb each) T-bone steaks
- 1 tablespoon olive oil
- 1 tablespoon sea salt
- 1 teaspoon black pepper
- 1 teaspoon garlic powder

Directions:
1. Preheat your grill to high heat.
2. Brush the T-bone steaks with olive oil and season with sea salt, black pepper, and garlic powder on both sides.
3. Place the steaks on the grill and cook for 6-8 minutes per side, or until they reach your desired level of doneness. Use a meat thermometer to check for an internal temperature of 135°F (57°C) for medium-rare.
4. Remove the steaks from the grill and let them rest for 5-10 minutes before serving.

Number of servings: 2

Preparation time: 10 minutes

Cooking time: 15 minutes

Nutritional value per serving:
Calories: 650, Carbs: 1g, Fiber: 0g, Sugars: 0g, Protein: 65g, Saturated fat: 20g, Unsaturated fat: 28g

Difficulty rating: ★★☆☆

Tips for ingredient variations: For an extra kick, add 1 teaspoon of crushed red pepper flakes to the seasoning mix.

Chuck Roast with Bone Broth Gravy

Number of servings: 6

Preparation time: 15 minutes

Cooking time: 4 hours

Nutritional value per serving:
Calories: 480, Carbs: 3g, Fiber: 1g, Sugars: 1g, Protein: 45g, Saturated fat: 15g, Unsaturated fat: 20g

Difficulty rating: ★★★☆☆

Tips for ingredient variations: Add 1 cup of chopped carrots and celery to the pot for extra flavor and nutrients.

Directions:
1. Preheat your oven to 300°F (150°C).
2. In a large Dutch oven, heat the olive oil over medium-high heat.
3. Season the chuck roast with sea salt and black pepper, then brown it on all sides in the Dutch oven. Remove and set aside.
4. Add the chopped onion and minced garlic to the pot, sautéing until soft and fragrant.
5. Stir in the tomato paste and cook for 1 minute.
6. Pour in the beef bone broth, scraping up any browned bits from the bottom of the pot.
7. Put the fresh rosemary back in the pot with the chuck roast.
8. Cover and roast in the oven for 4 hours, or until the meat is tender and easily shredded.
9. Remove the rosemary sprigs and shred the roast before serving with the gravy.

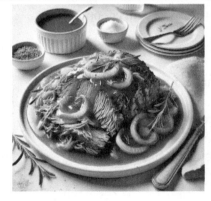

Ingredients:
- 3 lbs chuck roast
- 2 tablespoons olive oil
- 1 cup beef bone broth
- 1 onion, chopped
- 2 cloves garlic, minced
- 1 tablespoon tomato paste
- 1 teaspoon sea salt
- ½ teaspoon black pepper
- 2 sprigs fresh rosemary

Beef and Liver Burgers

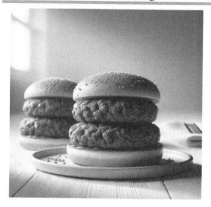

Ingredients:

• 1 lb ground beef
• ½ lb beef liver, finely chopped or ground
• 1 egg
• 2 cloves garlic, minced
• 1 teaspoon onion powder
• Sea salt and black pepper to taste
• 2 tablespoons butter

Directions:

1. In a large bowl, combine the ground beef, chopped liver, egg, garlic, onion powder, sea salt, and black pepper. Stir thoroughly to ensure that all ingredients are combined equally.
2. Create four equal-sized patties out of the mixture.
3. Heat a skillet over medium-high heat and melt the butter.
4. Cook the patties in the skillet for about 6-7 minutes per side, or until they reach your desired level of doneness.
5. Before serving, take the patties out of the skillet and rest them for a few minutes.

Number of servings: 4

Preparation time: 20 minutes

Cooking time: 15 minutes

Nutritional value per serving:
Calories: 310, Carbs: 2g, Fiber: 0g, Sugars: 0g, Protein: 28g, Saturated fat: 10g, Unsaturated fat: 12g

Difficulty rating: ★★☆☆

Tips for ingredient variations: Add 1 tablespoon of Worcestershire sauce for additional flavor.

Spicy Beef Tongue Tacos (Carnivore Style)

Number of servings: 4

Preparation time: 30 minutes (plus overnight marinating)

Cooking time: 3 hours

Nutritional value per serving:
Calories: 270, Carbs: 1g, Fiber: 0g, Sugars: 0g, Protein: 32g, Saturated fat: 10g, Unsaturated fat: 15g

Difficulty rating: ★★★☆☆

Tips for ingredient variations: Add a dollop of sour cream or shredded cheese to each taco wrap for extra flavor.

Directions:

1. Clean the beef tongue and marinate it overnight in a mixture of sea salt, black pepper, smoked paprika, cayenne pepper, garlic, and olive oil.
2. The next day, preheat your oven to 300°F (150°C).
3. Place the beef tongue in a roasting pan and cover it with foil.
4. Roast for 3 hours or until the tongue is tender.
5. Let the tongue cool slightly, then peel off the outer layer of skin.
6. Slice the tongue thinly and serve in large lettuce leaves as taco wraps.

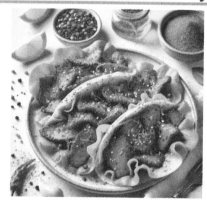

Ingredients:

• 1 beef tongue
• 2 tablespoons coarse sea salt
• 1 tablespoon black pepper
• 1 tablespoon smoked paprika
• 1 teaspoon cayenne pepper
• 2 cloves garlic, minced
• 1 tablespoon olive oil
• 8 large lettuce leaves (for wrapping)

Venison Stew

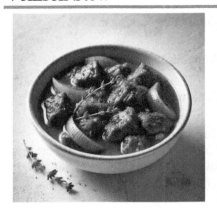

Ingredients:

- 2 lbs venison, cubed
- 4 tablespoons butter
- 1 large onion, diced
- 3 cloves garlic, minced
- 4 cups bone broth
- 2 bay leaves
- 1 teaspoon dried thyme
- Sea salt and black pepper to taste

Directions:

1. In a large pot, melt the butter over medium heat. Cook the minced garlic and onion until they become tender.
2. Add the cubed venison to the pot, searing on all sides until browned.
3. Pour in the bone broth and add the bay leaves, thyme, sea salt, and black pepper.
4. Bring the mixture to a boil, then reduce heat and let it simmer for about 2 hours, or until the venison is tender.
5. Remove the bay leaves before serving.

Number of servings: 6

Preparation time: 15 minutes

Cooking time: 2 hours

Nutritional value per serving:
Calories: 320, Carbs: 3g, Fiber: 0g, Sugars: 1g, Protein: 40g, Saturated fat: 10g, Unsaturated fat: 14g

Difficulty rating: ★★☆☆

Tips for ingredient variations: For a richer flavor, add 1 cup of red wine to the stew during the cooking process.

Garlic Herb Prime Rib

Number of servings: 6

Preparation time: 20 minutes

Cooking time: 2 hours

Nutritional value per serving:
Calories: 700, Carbs: 2g, Fiber: 0g, Sugars: 0g, Protein: 60g, Saturated fat: 25g, Unsaturated fat: 35g

Difficulty rating: ★★★☆☆

Tips for ingredient variations: Add 1 teaspoon of smoked paprika to the spice mixture for an extra depth of flavor.

Directions:

1. Preheat your oven to 450°F (230°C).
2. In a small bowl, mix together the sea salt, black pepper, minced garlic, rosemary, and thyme.
3. Rub the spice mixture all over the prime rib roast, ensuring it is evenly coated.
4. Put the roast, fat side up, on a rack inside a roasting pan.
5. Roast for 15 minutes, then reduce the oven temperature to 325°F (165°C) and continue cooking for about 1 hour and 45 minutes, or until the internal temperature reaches 135°F (57°C) for medium-rare.
6. Baste the roast with the melted butter halfway through the cooking time.
7. Remove the roast from the oven and let it rest for 15 minutes before slicing.

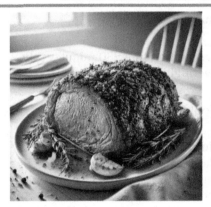

Ingredients:

- 1 (4 lb) prime rib roast
- 3 tablespoons coarse sea salt
- 2 tablespoons black pepper
- 2 tablespoons minced garlic
- 1 tablespoon dried rosemary
- 1 tablespoon dried thyme
- 4 tablespoons butter, melted

Beef Shank Osso Buco

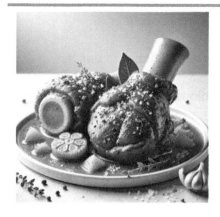

Ingredients:
- 4 beef shanks (about 1.5 inches thick)
- 1 teaspoon sea salt
- 1 teaspoon black pepper
- 4 tablespoons butter
- 1 large onion, diced
- 3 cloves garlic, minced
- 2 cups bone broth
- 1 cup dry white wine
- 2 bay leaves
- 1 teaspoon dried thyme

Directions:
1. Season the beef shanks with sea salt and black pepper.
2. In a large ovenproof pot, melt the butter over medium-high heat. Sear the beef shanks on all sides until browned. Remove and set aside.
3. Add the diced onion and minced garlic to the pot, cooking until softened.
4. Return the beef shanks to the pot and pour in the bone broth and white wine. Add the bay leaves and thyme.
5. Bring the mixture to a simmer, then cover and transfer the pot to an oven preheated to 325°F (165°C).
6. Cook for 2-2.5 hours, or until the meat is tender and falling off the bone.
7. Remove the bay leaves before serving.

Number of servings: 4

Preparation time: 20 minutes

Cooking time: 2.5 hours

Nutritional value per serving:
Calories: 450, Carbs: 3g, Fiber: 0g, Sugars: 1g, Protein: 45g, Saturated fat: 20g, Unsaturated fat: 15g

Difficulty rating: ★★★☆☆

Tips for ingredient variations: Garnish with fresh parsley and lemon zest before serving for a burst of freshness.

Veal Cutlets with Lemon Butter Sauce

Number of servings: 4

Preparation time: 10 minutes

Cooking time: 20 minutes

Nutritional value per serving:
Calories: 300, Carbs: 2g, Fiber: 0g, Sugars: 0g, Protein: 36g, Saturated fat: 6g, Unsaturated fat: 10g

Difficulty rating: ★★☆☆☆

Tips for ingredient variations: For an extra flavor boost, add a splash of white wine to the sauce before returning the veal cutlets to the skillet.

Directions:
1. Season the veal cutlets with sea salt and black pepper on both sides.
2. In a large skillet, melt the butter over medium-high heat.
3. Add the veal cutlets to the skillet and cook for 3-4 minutes on each side, until golden brown and cooked through. Remove the cutlets from the skillet and set aside.
4. In the same skillet, add the lemon juice, lemon zest, and capers. Cook for 1-2 minutes, stirring occasionally.
5. Spoon the sauce over the veal cutlets and return them to the stove. Cook for an additional 1-2 minutes.
6. Sprinkle with fresh parsley before serving warm.

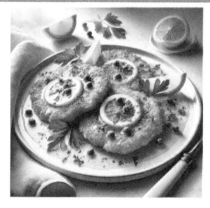

Ingredients:
- 4 veal cutlets
- 2 tablespoons butter
- 1 lemon, juiced and zested
- 1 tablespoon capers, drained
- 1 tablespoon fresh parsley, chopped
- Sea salt and black pepper to taste

Lamb Shoulder Roast

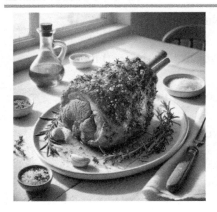

Ingredients:

- 1 (3-4 lb) lamb shoulder roast
- 3 cloves garlic, minced
- 2 tablespoons olive oil
- 2 teaspoons fresh rosemary, chopped
- 2 teaspoons fresh thyme, chopped
- Sea salt and black pepper to taste

Directions:

1. Preheat your oven to 325°F (165°C).
2. In a small bowl, combine the garlic, olive oil, rosemary, thyme, sea salt, and black pepper.
3. Rub the garlic and herb mixture all over the lamb shoulder roast, ensuring it is evenly coated.
4. After putting the lamb shoulder in a roasting pan, cover it with foil.
5. Roast in the preheated oven for 2 hours. Remove the foil and roast for an additional 30 minutes, or until the lamb is tender and has a golden brown crust.
6. Before slicing, take the lamb out of the oven and allow it to rest for ten to fifteen minutes.

Number of servings: 6

Preparation time: 15 minutes

Cooking time: 2 hours 30 minutes

Nutritional value per serving:
Calories: 450, Carbs: 1g, Fiber: 0g, Sugars: 0g, Protein: 42g, Saturated fat: 16g, Unsaturated fat: 20g

Difficulty rating: ★★★☆☆

Tips for ingredient variations: Add a splash of balsamic vinegar to the herb mixture for a slightly tangy flavor.

Bison Ribeye with Horseradish Cream

Number of servings: 4

Preparation time: 10 minutes

Cooking time: 20 minutes

Nutritional value per serving:
Calories: 500, Carbs: 2g, Fiber: 0g, Sugars: 1g, Protein: 48g, Saturated fat: 15g, Unsaturated fat: 18g

Difficulty rating: ★★★☆☆

Tips for ingredient variations: For a spicier kick, add a pinch of cayenne pepper to the horseradish cream.

Directions:

1. Preheat your grill to high heat.
2. Rub the bison ribeye steaks with olive oil, sea salt, and black pepper.
3. Cook the steaks for 4–5 minutes on each side, or until the doneness you desire is achieved. After taking the steaks off the grill, rest them for five minutes.
4. In a small bowl, combine the sour cream, prepared horseradish, lemon juice, and fresh chives. Mix well.
5. Serve the bison ribeye steaks with a dollop of horseradish cream on top.

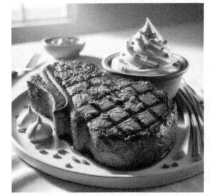

Ingredients:

- 4 bison ribeye steaks
- 2 tablespoons olive oil
- Sea salt and black pepper to taste
- ½ cup sour cream
- 2 tablespoons prepared horseradish
- 1 teaspoon lemon juice
- 1 tablespoon fresh chives, chopped

Roast Chicken with Herb Butter

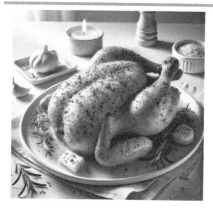

Ingredients:

• 1 whole chicken (about 4 lbs), giblets removed
• 1/2 cup butter, softened
• 2 tablespoons fresh rosemary, chopped
• 2 tablespoons fresh thyme, chopped
• 4 cloves garlic, minced
• Sea salt and black pepper to taste
• 1 lemon, halved

Directions:

1. Preheat your oven to 375°F (190°C).
2. In a small bowl, mix together the butter, rosemary, thyme, garlic, salt, and pepper until well combined.
3. Rub the herb butter mixture all over the chicken, including under the skin and inside the cavity.
4. Place the lemon halves inside the chicken cavity.
5. Tie the chicken legs together with kitchen twine and place the chicken breast-side up in a roasting pan.
6. Roast for one hour and thirty minutes, or until the skin is crispy and golden and the interior temperature reaches 165°F (74°C).
7. Let the chicken rest for 10 minutes before carving and serving.

Number of servings: 6

Preparation time: 15 minutes

Cooking time: 1 hour 30 minutes

Nutritional value per serving: Calories: 450, Carbs: 1g, Fiber: 0g, Sugars: 0g, Protein: 35g, Saturated fat: 14g, Unsaturated fat: 18g

Difficulty rating: ★★★☆☆

Tips for ingredient variations: Add a splash of white wine or chicken broth to the roasting pan for added moisture and flavor.

Duck Breast with Crispy Skin

Number of servings: 4

Preparation time: 10 minutes

Cooking time: 25 minutes

Nutritional value per serving: Calories: 360, Carbs: 0g, Fiber: 0g, Sugars: 0g, Protein: 30g, Saturated fat: 8g, Unsaturated fat: 16g

Difficulty rating: ★★★☆☆

Tips for ingredient variations: Serve with a side of sautéed spinach or roasted Brussels sprouts for a complete meal.

Directions:

1. Preheat your oven to 400°F (200°C).
2. Score the skin of the duck breasts in a crosshatch pattern, being careful not to cut into the meat.
3. Season both sides of the duck breasts with salt, pepper, garlic powder, and thyme.
4. Place the duck breasts skin-side down in a cold, oven-safe skillet. After the skin is crispy and golden brown, reduce the heat to medium and cook for 8 to 10 minutes.
5. Flip the duck breasts over and transfer the skillet to the oven.
6. Roast for 6-10 minutes, or until the internal temperature reaches 135°F (57°C) for medium-rare.
7. Let the duck breasts rest for 5 minutes before slicing and serving.

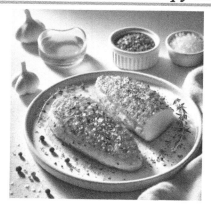

Ingredients:

• 4 duck breasts, skin on
• Sea salt and black pepper to taste
• 1 teaspoon garlic powder
• 1 teaspoon dried thyme

Chicken Thighs in Cream Sauce

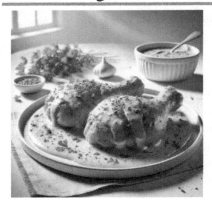

Ingredients:

• 8 chicken thighs, skin on
• Sea salt and black pepper to taste
• 2 tablespoons butter
• 1 cup heavy cream
• 1/2 cup chicken broth
• 1 tablespoon Dijon mustard
• 4 cloves garlic, minced
• 2 tablespoons fresh parsley, chopped

Directions:

1. Preheat your oven to 375°F (190°C).
2. Season the chicken thighs with salt and pepper.
3. In a large oven-safe skillet, melt the butter over medium-high heat. After placing the chicken thighs skin-side down, roast them for five to seven minutes, or until the skin is crispy and golden. Flip the thighs and cook for another 5 minutes.
4. After taking the chicken out of the skillet, set it aside.
5. Add the garlic to the same skillet and sauté for 1 minute, or until fragrant. Stir in the heavy cream, chicken broth, and Dijon mustard, scraping up any browned bits from the bottom of the skillet.
6. Spoon some of the sauce over the chicken thighs and return them to the skillet, skin-side up.
7. Transfer the skillet to the oven and bake for 30 minutes, or until the chicken is cooked through and the sauce has thickened.
8. Garnish with chopped parsley before serving.

Number of servings: 4

Preparation time: 10 minutes

Cooking time: 45 minutes

Nutritional value per serving: Calories: 520, Carbs: 2g, Fiber: 0g, Sugars: 1g, Protein: 36g, Saturated fat: 24g, Unsaturated fat: 12g

Difficulty rating:
★★☆☆

Tips for ingredient variations: Add mushrooms or spinach to the cream sauce for additional flavor and nutrients.

Bacon-Wrapped Chicken Breasts

Number of servings: 4

Preparation time: 10 minutes

Cooking time: 30 minutes

Nutritional value per serving:
Calories: 360, Carbs: 1g, Fiber: 0g, Sugars: 0g, Protein: 40g, Saturated fat: 10g, Unsaturated fat: 14g

Difficulty rating: ★★☆☆

Tips for ingredient variations: Add a slice of cheese inside the chicken breast before wrapping with bacon for an extra layer of flavor.

Directions:

1. Preheat your oven to 375°F (190°C).
2. Season the chicken breasts with salt, pepper, garlic powder, and paprika.
3. Use toothpicks to secure the two bacon strips around each chicken breast.
4. Place the bacon-wrapped chicken breasts on a baking sheet lined with parchment paper.
5. Bake for 25-30 minutes, or until the chicken is cooked through and the bacon is crispy.
6. Let the chicken rest for 5 minutes before serving.

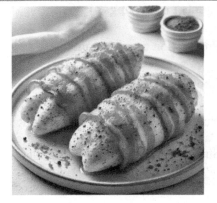

Ingredients:

• 4 chicken breasts
• 8 slices bacon
• Sea salt and black pepper to taste
• 1 teaspoon garlic powder
• 1 teaspoon paprika

Turkey Drumsticks with Garlic Butter

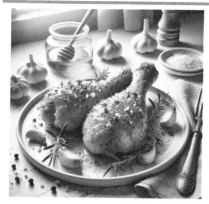

Ingredients:

• 4 turkey drumsticks
• Sea salt and black pepper to taste
• 4 tablespoons butter, melted
• 4 cloves garlic, minced
• 1 tablespoon fresh rosemary, chopped
• 1 tablespoon fresh thyme, chopped

Directions:

1. Preheat your oven to 350°F (175°C).
2. Season the turkey drumsticks with salt and pepper.
3. In a small bowl, mix together the melted butter, garlic, rosemary, and thyme.
4. Place the drumsticks in a roasting pan and brush with the garlic butter mixture.
5. Roast for 1 hour and 30 minutes, basting every 30 minutes, until the drumsticks are cooked through and the skin is crispy.
6. Let the drumsticks rest for 10 minutes before serving.

Number of servings: 4

Preparation time: 10 minutes

Cooking time: 1 hour 30 minutes

Nutritional value per serving:
Calories: 480, Carbs: 1g, Fiber: 0g, Sugars: 0g, Protein: 45g, Saturated fat: 12g, Unsaturated fat: 18g

Difficulty rating: ★★★☆☆

Tips for ingredient variations: Add a splash of lemon juice to the garlic butter for a fresh, zesty flavor.

Grilled Chicken Wings

Number of servings: 4

Preparation time: 10 minutes

Cooking time: 25 minutes

Nutritional value per serving:
Calories: 380, Carbs: 0g, Fiber: 0g, Sugars: 0g, Protein: 30g, Saturated fat: 6g, Unsaturated fat: 22g

Difficulty rating: ★★☆☆☆

Tips for ingredient variations: For extra flavor, marinate the wings in a mixture of olive oil, lemon juice, and fresh herbs for a few hours before grilling.

Directions:

1. Preheat your grill to medium-high heat.
2. Toss the chicken wings in a big bowl with olive oil, dried thyme, sea salt, black pepper, paprika, and garlic powder until well covered.
3. Place the chicken wings on the grill in a single layer.
4. The wings should be cooked through and crispy after 20 to 25 minutes on the grill, turning them over once or twice.
5. Before serving, remove from the grill and rest for a few minutes.

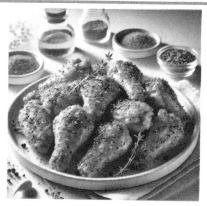

Ingredients:

• 2 lbs chicken wings
• 2 tablespoons olive oil
• 1 tablespoon garlic powder
• 1 teaspoon sea salt
• 1 teaspoon black pepper
• 1 teaspoon paprika
• 1 teaspoon dried thyme

Rabbit Stew

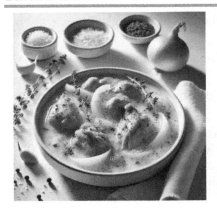

Ingredients:

- 1 whole rabbit, cut into pieces
- 3 tablespoons butter
- 1 large onion, chopped
- 3 cloves garlic, minced
- 1 cup bone broth
- 1 cup heavy cream
- 1 teaspoon dried thyme
- 1 teaspoon sea salt
- 1 teaspoon black pepper

Directions:

1. In a large pot, melt the butter over medium heat. Add the rabbit pieces and brown on all sides.
2. Remove the rabbit from the pot and set aside.
3. Add the minced garlic and diced onion to the pot and sauté until aromatic and tender.
4. Return the rabbit to the pot and add the bone broth, heavy cream, dried thyme, sea salt, and black pepper.
5. Bring to a boil, then reduce the heat to low and simmer for 2 hours, or until the rabbit is tender.
6. Serve the stew hot.

Number of servings: 4

Preparation time: 20 minutes

Cooking time: 2 hours

Nutritional value per serving:
Calories: 480, Carbs: 3g, Fiber: 0g, Sugars: 1g, Protein: 38g, Saturated fat: 18g, Unsaturated fat: 12g

Difficulty rating: ★★★☆☆

Tips for ingredient variations: Add a splash of white wine for extra depth of flavor.

Pheasant Breast with Mustard Sauce

Number of servings: 4

Preparation time: 10 minutes

Cooking time: 20 minutes

Nutritional value per serving:
Calories: 430, Carbs: 2g, Fiber: 0g, Sugars: 1g, Protein: 32g, Saturated fat: 18g, Unsaturated fat: 12g

Difficulty rating: ★★☆☆☆

Tips for ingredient variations: Garnish with fresh parsley or chives for a burst of color and flavor.

Directions:

1. Melt the butter in a big skillet over medium heat.
2. Season the pheasant breasts with sea salt and black pepper, then add to the skillet. Cook for 5-7 minutes per side, until browned and cooked through.
3. Remove the pheasant breasts from the skillet and set aside.
4. Add the heavy cream, Dijon mustard, and dried tarragon to the skillet, stirring to combine. Simmer the sauce for three to four minutes, or until it thickens.
5. Return the pheasant breasts to the skillet and coat with the mustard sauce. Cook for an additional 2-3 minutes.
6. Serve the pheasant breasts with the mustard sauce drizzled on top.

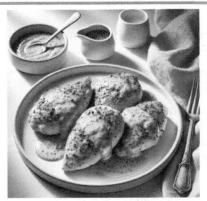

Ingredients:

- 4 pheasant breasts
- 2 tablespoons butter
- 1 cup heavy cream
- 2 tablespoons Dijon mustard
- 1 teaspoon sea salt
- 1 teaspoon black pepper
- 1 teaspoon dried tarragon

Slow-Cooked Duck Legs

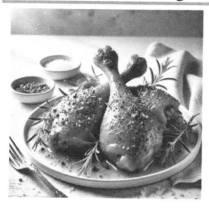

Ingredients:
- 4 duck legs with thighs
- 2 tablespoons olive oil
- 4 cloves garlic, minced
- 1 teaspoon sea salt
- 1 teaspoon black pepper
- 1 teaspoon dried rosemary
- 1 cup bone broth

Directions:
1. Preheat your oven to 300°F (150°C).
2. In a large oven-safe pot, heat the olive oil over medium-high heat. Add the duck legs and brown on all sides.
3. Remove the duck legs from the pot and set aside.
4. Add the minced garlic to the pot and sauté until fragrant.
5. Return the duck legs to the pot and season with sea salt, black pepper, and dried rosemary.
6. Pour the bone broth over the duck legs.
7. Cover the pot and transfer to the preheated oven. Cook the duck legs slowly for three hours, or until they are soft.
8. Serve the duck legs with the cooking juices.

Number of servings: 4

Preparation time: 15 minutes

Cooking time: 3 hours

Nutritional value per serving:
Calories: 520, Carbs: 1g, Fiber: 0g, Sugars: 0g, Protein: 40g, Saturated fat: 14g, Unsaturated fat: 26g

Difficulty rating: ★★★☆☆

Tips for ingredient variations: Add a splash of red wine for a richer flavor profile.

Chicken Alfredo (Carnivore Style)

Number of servings: 4

Preparation time: 15 minutes

Cooking time: 25 minutes

Nutritional value per serving:
Calories: 600, Carbs: 3g, Fiber: 0g, Sugars: 1g, Protein: 45g, Saturated fat: 28g, Unsaturated fat: 14g

Difficulty rating: ★★☆☆☆

Tips for ingredient variations: Add a pinch of nutmeg to the Alfredo sauce for a subtle, warm flavor.

Directions:
1. In a large skillet, melt the butter over medium-high heat. Add the chicken breasts and cook for 5 to 7 minutes on each side, or slow-cook for 3 hours, until browned and cooked through. Remove from the skillet and set aside.
2. Reduce the heat to medium and add the minced garlic to the skillet. Sauté until fragrant.
3. Pour in the heavy cream and bring to a simmer.
4. Stir in the grated Parmesan cheese, sea salt, and black pepper. Cook until the sauce thickens.
5. Pour the Alfredo sauce over the chicken breasts and place them back in the skillet. Cook for an additional 2-3 minutes.
6. Serve the chicken Alfredo hot.

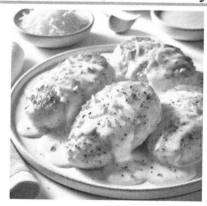

Ingredients:
- 4 boneless, skinless chicken breasts
- 2 tablespoons butter
- 1 cup heavy cream
- 1 cup grated Parmesan cheese
- 2 cloves garlic, minced
- 1 teaspoon sea salt
- 1 teaspoon black pepper

Goose Breast with Red Wine Reduction

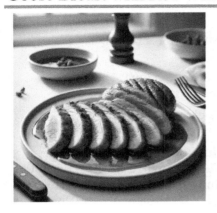

Ingredients:

• 4 goose breasts
• 2 tablespoons olive oil
• Sea salt and black pepper to taste
• 1 cup red wine
• 1 cup beef broth
• 2 cloves garlic, minced
• 1 sprig fresh rosemary

Directions:

1. Preheat your oven to 375°F (190°C).
2. Heat olive oil in a large oven-safe skillet over medium-high heat. Season goose breasts with salt and pepper.
3. Sear the goose breasts in the skillet, skin side down, for 4-5 minutes until the skin is crispy. For a further two to three minutes, flip and sear the other side.
4. Transfer the skillet to the oven and roast for 20-25 minutes or until the internal temperature reaches 135°F (57°C) for medium-rare.
5. Remove the goose breasts from the skillet and let them rest while you prepare the reduction.
6. In the same skillet, add minced garlic and rosemary, and cook over medium heat until fragrant.
7. Pour in the red wine and beef broth, scraping up any browned bits from the bottom of the skillet. Simmer until the liquid reduces by half, about 10 minutes.
8. Slice the goose breasts and serve with the red wine reduction drizzled on top.

Number of servings: 4

Preparation time: 15 minutes

Cooking time: 45 minutes

Nutritional value per serving: Calories: 390, Carbs: 2g, Fiber: 0g, Sugars: 1g, Protein: 35g, Saturated fat: 8g, Unsaturated fat: 12g

Difficulty rating:
★★★☆☆

Tips for ingredient variations: Add a tablespoon of honey to the reduction for a touch of sweetness.

Lemon Garlic Chicken Skewers

Number of servings: 4

Preparation time: 15 minutes

Cooking time: 20 minutes

Nutritional value per serving:
Calories: 210, Carbs: 2g, Fiber: 0g, Sugars: 0g, Protein: 28g, Saturated fat: 2g, Unsaturated fat: 8g

Difficulty rating: ★★☆☆☆

Tips for ingredient variations: Add a pinch of red pepper flakes to the marinade for a spicy kick.

Directions:

1. Mix the lemon zest, juice, olive oil, minced garlic, salt, and pepper in a big bowl. Add the chicken cubes and toss to coat. Marinate for at least 30 minutes.
2. Preheat your grill to medium-high heat.
3. Thread the marinated chicken cubes onto skewers.
4. Grill the skewers for 10-15 minutes, turning occasionally, until the chicken is fully cooked and slightly charred.
5. Sprinkle with fresh parsley before serving.

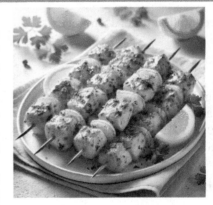

Ingredients:

• 1 pound chicken breasts, cut into cubes
• 2 lemons, juiced and zested
• 3 cloves garlic, minced
• 2 tablespoons olive oil
• Sea salt and black pepper to taste
• 2 tablespoons fresh parsley, chopped

Pork Tenderloin with Apple Reduction

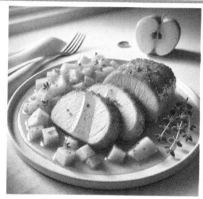

Ingredients:

• 1 (1.5 lb) pork tenderloin
• Sea salt and black pepper to taste
• 2 tablespoons olive oil
• 2 apples, peeled and diced
• 1 cup apple cider
• 1 tablespoon apple cider vinegar
• 1 teaspoon fresh thyme, chopped

Directions:

1. Preheat your oven to 375°F (190°C).
2. Season the pork tenderloin with salt and pepper.
3. In a skillet that is ovensafe, warm the olive oil over medium-high heat. The pork tenderloin should sear for four to five minutes, or until browned on all sides.
4. Transfer the skillet to the oven and roast for 20-25 minutes, or until the internal temperature reaches 145°F (63°C).
5. Remove the tenderloin from the skillet and let it rest while you prepare the apple reduction.
6. In the same skillet, add the diced apples and cook over medium heat until softened, about 5 minutes.
7. Pour in the apple cider and apple cider vinegar, scraping up any browned bits from the bottom of the skillet. Simmer until the liquid reduces by half, about 10 minutes.
8. Slice the pork tenderloin and serve with the apple reduction spooned over the top, garnished with fresh thyme.

Number of servings: 4

Preparation time: 15 minutes

Cooking time: 30 minutes

Nutritional value per serving: Calories: 320, Carbs: 12g, Fiber: 2g, Sugars: 10g, Protein: 28g, Saturated fat: 4g, Unsaturated fat: 10g

Difficulty rating:
★★☆☆

Tips for ingredient variations: Substitute pears for apples for a different flavor profile.

Stuffed Turkey Thighs

Number of servings: 4

Preparation time: 20 minutes

Cooking time: 1 hour 30 minutes

Nutritional value per serving: Calories: 450, Carbs: 2g, Fiber: 0g, Sugars: 0g, Protein: 50g, Saturated fat: 10g, Unsaturated fat: 12g

Difficulty rating: ★★★☆☆

Tips for ingredient variations: Add chopped spinach to the stuffing mixture for extra flavor and nutrients.

Directions:

1. Preheat your oven to 375°F (190°C).
2. In a bowl, combine ground pork, parmesan cheese, parsley, garlic, salt, and pepper.
3. Lay out the turkey thighs flat and spoon the pork mixture onto each thigh. Using kitchen twine, bind the thighs after rolling them up.
4. In an oven-safe skillet, warm the olive oil over medium-high heat. Sear the stuffed turkey thighs on all sides until browned, about 8-10 minutes.
5. Transfer the skillet to the oven and roast for 1 hour 20 minutes, or until the internal temperature reaches 165°F (74°C).
Remove the turkey thighs from the oven and let them rest for 10 minutes before slicing.

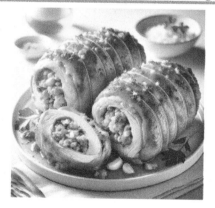

Ingredients:

• 4 turkey thighs, boned and skinned
• 1 pound ground pork
• 1/2 cup parmesan cheese, grated
• 1/4 cup fresh parsley, chopped
• 2 cloves garlic, minced
• Sea salt and black pepper to taste
2 tablespoons olive oil

6.

55

Chicken Liver Stroganoff

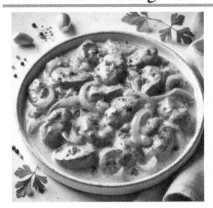

Ingredients:

- 1 pound chicken livers, cleaned and trimmed
- 2 tablespoons butter
- 1 onion, finely chopped
- 2 cloves garlic, minced
- 1 cup heavy cream
- 1 tablespoon Dijon mustard
- Sea salt and black pepper to taste
- 1 teaspoon paprika
- Fresh parsley, chopped for garnish

Directions:

1. Heat the butter in a large skillet over medium heat. Add the chopped onion and simmer for about 5 minutes, or until transparent.
2. Add the minced garlic and cook for an additional 1 minute.
3. Increase the heat to medium-high and add the chicken livers. Cook, stirring occasionally, until the livers are browned and cooked through, about 8-10 minutes.
4. Reduce the heat to medium-low and stir in the heavy cream, Dijon mustard, salt, pepper, and paprika. Let the sauce simmer for five to seven minutes so that it thickens.
5. Serve the stroganoff hot, garnished with fresh parsley.

Number of servings: 4

Preparation time: 15 minutes

Cooking time: 30 minutes

Nutritional value per serving:
Calories: 320, Carbs: 5g, Fiber: 1g, Sugars: 2g, Protein: 28g, Saturated fat: 14g, Unsaturated fat: 10g

Difficulty rating: ★★☆☆

Tips for ingredient variations: Add a splash of brandy to the sauce for a richer flavor.

BBQ Chicken Drumsticks

Number of servings: 4

Preparation time: 10 minutes

Cooking time: 50 minutes

Nutritional value per serving:
Calories: 310, Carbs: 4g, Fiber: 0g, Sugars: 2g, Protein: 28g, Saturated fat: 4g, Unsaturated fat: 8g

Difficulty rating: ★★☆☆

Tips for ingredient variations: For a spicier kick, add 1 teaspoon of cayenne pepper to the spice mixture.

Directions:

1. Preheat your oven to 400°F (200°C).
2. In a large bowl, mix together the olive oil, sea salt, black pepper, smoked paprika, garlic powder, and onion powder.
3. Place the chicken drumsticks in the basin and toss to ensure that the spice mixture coats them uniformly.
4. Arrange the drumsticks on a baking sheet lined with parchment paper.
5. Bake in the preheated oven for 40 minutes, turning once halfway through, until the chicken is cooked through and the skin is crispy.
6. Brush the drumsticks with the BBQ sauce and return to the oven for an additional 10 minutes.
7. Serve warm.

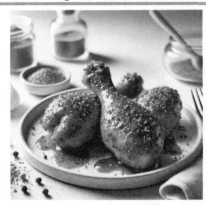

Ingredients:

- 8 chicken drumsticks
- 2 tablespoons olive oil
- 1 teaspoon sea salt
- 1 teaspoon black pepper
- 1 tablespoon smoked paprika
- 1 teaspoon garlic powder
- 1 teaspoon onion powder
- 1 cup sugar-free BBQ sauce

Pan-Seared Quail

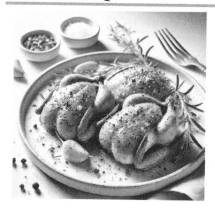

Ingredients:

- 8 quail, cleaned and patted dry
- 2 tablespoons olive oil
- 1 teaspoon sea salt
- 1 teaspoon black pepper
- 2 cloves garlic, minced
- 1 tablespoon fresh rosemary, chopped
- 1 tablespoon butter

Directions:

1. Season the quail with sea salt, black pepper, minced garlic, and chopped rosemary.
2. Heat the olive oil in a large skillet over medium-high heat.
3. Add the quail to the skillet and sear for about 4-5 minutes on each side, until golden brown and cooked through.
4. Reduce the heat to low and add the butter to the skillet. Spoon the melted butter over the quail to baste them.
5. Cook for an additional 2-3 minutes, ensuring the quail are fully cooked.
6. Serve warm.

Number of servings: 4

Preparation time: 10 minutes

Cooking time: 20 minutes

Nutritional value per serving: Calories: 250, Carbs: 0g, Fiber: 0g, Sugars: 0g, Protein: 20g, Saturated fat: 5g, Unsaturated fat: 10g

Difficulty rating: ★★☆☆

Tips for ingredient variations: For a citrus twist, add the juice of one lemon to the pan when basting the quail with butter.

Rabbit Sausage Patties

Number of servings: 4

Preparation time: 15 minutes

Cooking time: 15 minutes

Nutritional value per serving: Calories: 300, Carbs: 1g, Fiber: 0g, Sugars: 0g, Protein: 25g, Saturated fat: 7g, Unsaturated fat: 12g

Difficulty rating: ★★☆☆

Tips for ingredient variations: For added flavor, mix in 1/4 cup of finely chopped fresh herbs like parsley or thyme into the meat mixture before forming the patties.

Directions:

1. In a large bowl, mix together the ground rabbit meat, ground pork, sea salt, black pepper, fennel seeds, dried sage, garlic powder, and onion powder until well combined.
2. Form the mixture into 8 small patties.
3. In a big skillet, heat the olive oil over medium heat.
4. Add the sausage patties to the skillet and cook for about 6-8 minutes on each side, until golden brown and cooked through.
5. Serve warm.

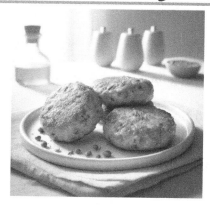

Ingredients:

- 1 lb ground rabbit meat
- 1/2 lb ground pork
- 1 teaspoon sea salt
- 1 teaspoon black pepper
- 1 teaspoon fennel seeds
- 1 teaspoon dried sage
- 1/2 teaspoon garlic powder
- 1/2 teaspoon onion powder
- 2 tablespoons olive oil

Butter-Basted Lobster Tails

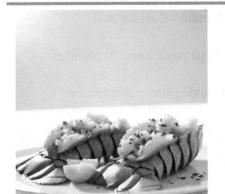

Ingredients:
- 4 lobster tails
- 1/2 cup butter, melted
- 2 cloves garlic, minced
- 1 tablespoon fresh lemon juice
- Sea salt and black pepper to taste
- Fresh parsley, chopped, for garnish

Directions:
1. Preheat your oven to 425°F (220°C).
2. Using kitchen shears, cut the top shell of the lobster tails lengthwise down the middle and pull the shells apart slightly to expose the meat.
3. In a small bowl, mix the melted butter, minced garlic, and lemon juice.
4. Place the lobster tails on a baking sheet and brush the butter mixture over the meat. Season with sea salt and black pepper.
5. Bake in the preheated oven for 12-15 minutes, or until the lobster meat is opaque and cooked through.
6. Add some chopped parsley as a garnish, then serve right away.

Number of servings: 4

Preparation time: 10 minutes

Cooking time: 15 minutes

Nutritional value per serving:
Calories: 290, Carbs: 2g, Fiber: 0g, Sugars: 0g, Protein: 28g, Saturated fat: 14g, Unsaturated fat: 10g

Difficulty rating: ★★☆☆

Tips for ingredient variations: Add a pinch of paprika to the butter mixture for a smoky flavor.

Garlic Shrimp Scampi

Number of servings: 4

Preparation time: 10 minutes

Cooking time: 10 minutes

Nutritional value per serving:
Calories: 210, Carbs: 2g, Fiber: 0g, Sugars: 0g, Protein: 24g, Saturated fat: 9g, Unsaturated fat: 7g

Difficulty rating: ★★☆☆

Tips for ingredient variations: Add a pinch of red pepper flakes for a spicy kick.

Directions:
1. Heat a large skillet over medium heat to melt butter.
2. Once aromatic, add the minced garlic and sauté for one to two minutes.
3. When the shrimp are pink and opaque, add them to the skillet and cook for two to three minutes on each side.
4. Pour in the chicken broth and lemon juice, bringing the mixture to a simmer.
5. Season with sea salt and black pepper to taste.
6. Remove from heat, garnish with chopped parsley, and serve warm.

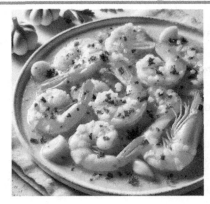

Ingredients:
- 1 lb shrimp, peeled and deveined
- 4 tablespoons butter
- 4 cloves garlic, minced
- 1/4 cup chicken broth
- 1/4 cup lemon juice
- Sea salt and black pepper to taste
1 tablespoon fresh parsley, chopped

Pan-Seared Scallops with Lemon Butter

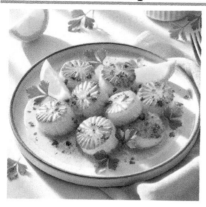

Ingredients:

• 1 lb sea scallops
• Sea salt and black pepper to taste
• 4 tablespoons butter
• 1 clove garlic, minced
• 2 tablespoons fresh lemon juice
• Fresh parsley, chopped, for garnish

Directions:

1. Pat the scallops dry with paper towels and season both sides with sea salt and black pepper.
2. Heat 2 tablespoons of butter in a large skillet over medium-high heat.
3. Add the scallops to the skillet and cook for 2-3 minutes on each side, until a golden crust forms and the scallops are opaque.
4. Remove the scallops from the skillet and set aside.
5. Reduce the heat to medium and add the remaining 2 tablespoons of butter and minced garlic to the skillet. Sauté for 1 minute until fragrant.
6. Stir in the lemon juice and cook for an additional minute.
7. Pour the lemon butter sauce over the scallops, garnish with chopped parsley, and serve immediately.

Number of servings: 4

Preparation time: 10 minutes

Cooking time: 10 minutes

Nutritional value per serving:
Calories: 210, Carbs: 1g, Fiber: 0g, Sugars: 0g, Protein: 19g, Saturated fat: 9g, Unsaturated fat: 7g

Difficulty rating: ★★☆☆☆

Tips for ingredient variations: Add a splash of white wine to the lemon butter sauce for extra flavor.

Grilled Swordfish Steaks

Number of servings: 4

Preparation time: 10 minutes

Cooking time: 10 minutes

Nutritional value per serving:
Calories: 250, Carbs: 1g, Fiber: 0g, Sugars: 0g, Protein: 30g, Saturated fat: 2g, Unsaturated fat: 10g

Difficulty rating: ★★☆☆☆

Tips for ingredient variations:
Marinate the swordfish in lemon juice, garlic, and herbs for 30 minutes before grilling for enhanced flavor.

Directions:

1. Preheat the grill to medium-high heat.
2. Brush the swordfish steaks with olive oil and season with sea salt and black pepper.
3. Grill the swordfish steaks for 4-5 minutes per side, until the fish is opaque and flakes easily with a fork.
4. Remove the steaks from the grill and drizzle with fresh lemon juice.
5. Garnish with chopped parsley and serve warm.

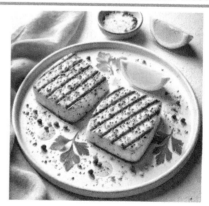

Ingredients:

• 4 swordfish steaks (6-8 oz each)
• 2 tablespoons olive oil
• Sea salt and black pepper to taste
• 1 tablespoon fresh lemon juice
• 1 tablespoon fresh parsley, chopped

Salmon Fillet with Dill Sauce

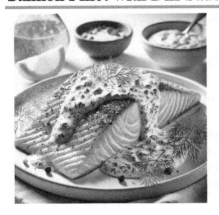

Ingredients:

- 4 salmon fillets (6 oz each)
- Sea salt and black pepper to taste
- 2 tablespoons olive oil
- 1/4 cup sour cream
- 1 tablespoon fresh dill, chopped
- 1 tablespoon lemon juice

Directions:

1. Preheat the oven to 400°F (200°C).
2. Season the salmon fillets with sea salt and black pepper.
3. In a large ovenproof skillet, heat the olive oil over medium-high heat.
4. Place the skin-side down salmon fillets on top and cook for 3–4 minutes, or until the skin is crispy.
5. Transfer the skillet to the preheated oven and bake for 8-10 minutes, until the salmon is cooked through.
6. Combine the sour cream, lemon juice, and chopped dill in a small bowl.
7. Serve the salmon fillets with the dill sauce on top.

Number of servings: 4

Preparation time: 10 minutes

Cooking time: 15 minutes

Nutritional value per serving:
Calories: 310, Carbs: 2g, Fiber: 0g, Sugars: 1g, Protein: 25g, Saturated fat: 6g, Unsaturated fat: 12g

Difficulty rating: ★★☆☆

Tips for ingredient variations: Add a teaspoon of capers to the dill sauce for a tangy twist.

Crab Cakes (Carnivore Style)

Number of servings: 4

Preparation time: 15 minutes

Cooking time: 20 minutes

Nutritional value per serving:
Calories: 220, Carbs: 1g, Fiber: 0g, Sugars: 0g, Protein: 20g, Saturated fat: 8g, Unsaturated fat: 5g

Difficulty rating: ★★☆☆

Tips for ingredient variations: For an extra kick, add a pinch of cayenne pepper to the crab mixture.

Directions:

1. In a large bowl, combine the crab meat, beaten eggs, crushed pork rinds, mayonnaise, Dijon mustard, lemon juice, Old Bay seasoning, sea salt, and black pepper.
2. Blend thoroughly until every component is combined equally.
3. Form the mixture into 8 patties.
4. In a large skillet over medium heat, melt the butter.
5. Cook the crab cakes for 4-5 minutes on each side, or until golden brown and cooked through.
6. Serve warm.

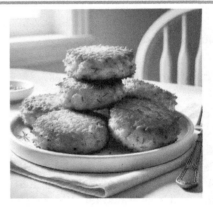

Ingredients:

- 1 lb crab meat, drained and picked over
- 2 large eggs, beaten
- ¼ cup pork rinds, crushed
- 2 tablespoons mayonnaise
- 1 tablespoon Dijon mustard
- 1 tablespoon lemon juice
- 1 teaspoon Old Bay seasoning
- Sea salt and black pepper to taste
- 2 tablespoons butter

Broiled Oysters with Herb Butter

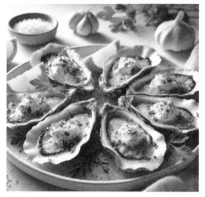

Ingredients:

• 24 oysters, shucked
• ½ cup butter, softened
• 2 cloves garlic, minced
• 2 tablespoons fresh parsley, chopped
• 1 tablespoon fresh chives, chopped
• 1 tablespoon lemon juice
• Sea salt and black pepper to taste

Directions:

1. Preheat your broiler to high.
2. In a small bowl, combine the softened butter, garlic, parsley, chives, lemon juice, sea salt, and black pepper. Mix until well blended.
3. Place the oysters on a baking sheet.
4. Spoon a small amount of herb butter onto each oyster.
5. Broil the oysters for 5-6 minutes, or until the butter is bubbling and the oysters are cooked through.
6. Serve immediately.

Number of servings: 4

Preparation time: 10 minutes

Cooking time: 10 minutes

Nutritional value per serving:
Calories: 180, Carbs: 2g, Fiber: 0g, Sugars: 0g, Protein: 10g, Saturated fat: 10g, Unsaturated fat: 5g

Difficulty rating: ★★☆☆☆

Tips for ingredient variations: Add a dash of hot sauce to the herb butter for a spicy twist.

Smoked Mackerel

Number of servings: 4

Preparation time: 10 minutes (plus 2 hours marinating time)

Cooking time: 1 hour

Nutritional value per serving:
Calories: 250, Carbs: 0g, Fiber: 0g, Sugars: 0g, Protein: 20g, Saturated fat: 2g, Unsaturated fat: 10g

Difficulty rating: ★★★☆☆

Tips for ingredient variations: Add wood chips like applewood or hickory to the smoker for enhanced flavor.

Directions:

1. In a large bowl, dissolve the sea salt and sugar in the water to create a brine.
2. Submerge the mackerel in the brine and refrigerate for 2 hours.
3. Preheat your smoker to 225°F (110°C).
4. Remove the mackerel from the brine, rinse under cold water, and pat dry.
5. Brush the mackerel with olive oil and season with freshly ground black pepper.
6. Place the mackerel in the smoker and smoke for 1 hour, or until the fish flakes easily with a fork.
7. Serve warm or chilled.

Ingredients:

• 4 whole mackerel, cleaned and gutted
• ¼ cup sea salt
• ¼ cup sugar
• 4 cups water
• 2 tablespoons olive oil
• Freshly ground black pepper to taste

Tuna Steaks with Wasabi Butter

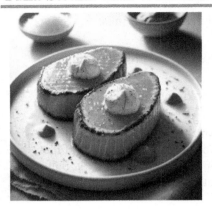

Ingredients:
- 4 tuna steaks (6-7 ounces each)
- 2 tablespoons olive oil
- Sea salt and black pepper to taste
- ½ cup butter, softened
- 1 tablespoon wasabi paste
- 1 teaspoon soy sauce (optional)

Directions:
1. Preheat your grill to high heat.
2. Brush the tuna steaks with olive oil and season with sea salt and black pepper.
3. In a small bowl, mix the softened butter, wasabi paste, and soy sauce (if using) until well combined.
4. Grill the tuna steaks for 3-4 minutes per side, or until desired doneness is reached.
5. Top each tuna steak with a dollop of wasabi butter just before serving.
6. Serve warm.

Number of servings: 4

Preparation time: 10 minutes

Cooking time: 10 minutes

Nutritional value per serving:
Calories: 300, Carbs: 1g, Fiber: 0g, Sugars: 0g, Protein: 30g, Saturated fat: 10g, Unsaturated fat: 12g

Difficulty rating: ★★☆☆

Tips for ingredient variations: Add finely chopped green onions to the wasabi butter for extra flavor and a bit of crunch.

Grilled Octopus with Olive Oil

Number of servings: 4

Preparation time: 15 minutes

Cooking time: 1 hour

Nutritional value per serving:
Calories: 200, Carbs: 2g, Fiber: 0g, Sugars: 0g, Protein: 20g, Saturated fat: 2g, Unsaturated fat: 14g

Difficulty rating: ★★★☆☆

Tips for ingredient variations:
Marinate the octopus in olive oil, garlic, and lemon juice for an hour before grilling for added flavor.

Directions:
1. In a large pot, combine the water, white wine, bay leaves, garlic, and lemon halves. Bring to a boil.
2. Add the octopus and reduce to a simmer. Cook for 45 minutes to 1 hour, or until the octopus is tender.
3. Preheat your grill to medium-high heat.
4. Remove the octopus from the pot and let it cool slightly. Cut into large pieces.
5. Brush the octopus with olive oil and season with sea salt and black pepper.
6. Grill the octopus for 2-3 minutes per side, or until charred and heated through.
7. Serve warm with a drizzle of olive oil.

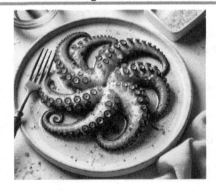

Ingredients:
- 2 lbs octopus, cleaned
- 4 cups water
- 1 cup white wine
- 2 bay leaves
- 4 cloves garlic, crushed
- 1 lemon, halved
- ¼ cup olive oil
- Sea salt and black pepper to taste

Grilled Ribeye Steak with Rosemary Butter

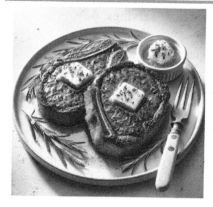

Ingredients:

• 4 ribeye steaks (about 8 ounces each)
• 2 tablespoons olive oil
• 4 cloves garlic, minced
• 2 teaspoons fresh rosemary, chopped
• Sea salt and black pepper to taste
• 4 tablespoons unsalted butter, softened
• 1 teaspoon lemon juice

Directions:

1. Preheat your grill to high heat.
2. In a small bowl, mix together the olive oil, minced garlic, chopped rosemary, sea salt, and black pepper.
3. Rub the ribeye steaks with the olive oil mixture, ensuring they are evenly coated.
4. Place the steaks on the preheated grill and cook for 4-5 minutes per side for medium-rare, or to your desired level of doneness.
5. While the steaks are grilling, combine the softened butter with the lemon juice in a small bowl.
6. Take the steaks off the grill after they are done and let them rest for a few minutes.
7. Top each steak with a dollop of the rosemary butter.
8. Serve warm with your favorite side dishes.

Number of servings: 4

Preparation time: 10 minutes

Cooking time: 15 minutes

Nutritional value per serving:
Calories: 450, Carbs: 1g, Fiber: 0g, Sugars: 0g, Protein: 38g, Saturated fat: 18g, Unsaturated fat: 14g

Difficulty rating: ★★☆☆

Tips for ingredient variations: Add a pinch of crushed red pepper flakes to the rosemary butter for a hint of heat.

Blackened Catfish

Number of servings: 4

Preparation time: 10 minutes

Cooking time: 15 minutes

Nutritional value per serving:
Calories: 250, Carbs: 2g, Fiber: 1g, Sugars: 0g, Protein: 35g, Saturated fat: 2g, Unsaturated fat: 10g

Difficulty rating: ★★☆☆

Tips for ingredient variations: Add 1 teaspoon of lemon juice to the fillets before baking for a tangy flavor.

Directions:

1. Preheat your oven to 400°F (200°C).
2. Combine the dried oregano, dried thyme, cayenne pepper, onion powder, garlic powder, black pepper, and smoked paprika in a small bowl.
3. Brush the catfish fillets with olive oil and rub the spice mixture evenly over both sides.
4. Arrange the fillets onto a parchment paper-lined baking sheet.
5. Bake the fish for 12 to 15 minutes, or until it flakes easily with a fork and is opaque.
6. Serve warm with a side of your choice.

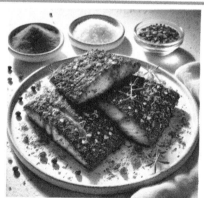

Ingredients:

• 4 catfish fillets
• 2 tablespoons olive oil
• 1 tablespoon smoked paprika
• 1 teaspoon garlic powder
• 1 teaspoon onion powder
• 1 teaspoon dried oregano
• 1 teaspoon dried thyme
• ½ teaspoon cayenne pepper
Sea salt and black pepper to taste

Shrimp and Crab Boil

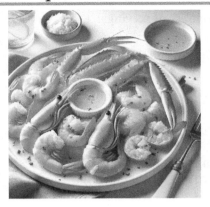

Ingredients:
- 1 lb shrimp, deveined and shells on
- 1 lb crab legs
- 4 cups water
- 1 lemon, halved
- 4 cloves garlic, smashed
- 2 tablespoons Old Bay seasoning
- 1 tablespoon sea salt
- 4 tablespoons butter, melted

Directions:
1. In a large pot, bring the water to a boil. Add the lemon halves, garlic, Old Bay seasoning, and sea salt.
2. Add the crab legs to the boiling water and cook for 10 minutes.
3. Add the shrimp and cook for an additional 5 minutes, or until the shrimp are pink and opaque.
4. Remove the pot from heat and drain the seafood, discarding the lemon and garlic.
5. Serve the shrimp and crab legs with melted butter for dipping.

Number of servings: 6

Preparation time: 20 minutes

Cooking time: 30 minutes

Nutritional value per serving:
Calories: 350, Carbs: 3g, Fiber: 0g, Sugars: 1g, Protein: 38g, Saturated fat: 10g, Unsaturated fat: 12g

Difficulty rating: ★★☆☆☆

Tips for ingredient variations: Add small red potatoes and corn on the cob for a more traditional boil.

Mussels in White Wine Sauce

Number of servings: 4

Preparation time: 10 minutes

Cooking time: 15 minutes

Nutritional value per serving:
Calories: 200, Carbs: 4g, Fiber: 0g, Sugars: 1g, Protein: 18g, Saturated fat: 5g, Unsaturated fat: 7g

Difficulty rating: ★★☆☆☆

Tips for ingredient variations: Add a pinch of red pepper flakes for a bit of heat.

Directions:
1. In a large pot, melt the butter over medium heat. Add the garlic and sauté until fragrant, about 1 minute.
2. Pour in the white wine and lemon juice, and bring to a simmer.
3. When the mussels have opened, add them to the pot, cover them, and cook for five to seven minutes.
4. If a mussel does not open, discard it.
5. Stir in the fresh parsley and season with sea salt and black pepper.
6. Serve the mussels in their broth with a side of crusty carnivore bread if desired.

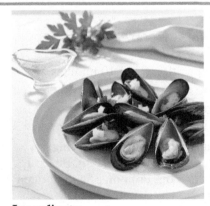

Ingredients:
- 2 lbs mussels, cleaned and debearded
- 2 tablespoons butter
- 4 cloves garlic, minced
- 1 cup dry white wine
- 1 lemon, juiced
- 2 tablespoons fresh parsley, chopped
- Sea salt and black pepper to taste

Sautéed Clams with Bacon

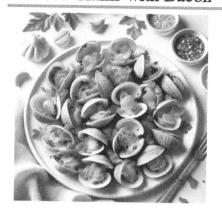

Ingredients:

- 2 lbs clams, cleaned
- 4 slices bacon, chopped
- 2 tablespoons butter
- 4 cloves garlic, minced
- 1/4 cup dry white wine
- 1 lemon, juiced
- Sea salt and black pepper to taste
- 2 tablespoons fresh parsley, chopped

Directions:

1. In a large skillet, cook the bacon over medium heat until crispy. Using a slotted spoon, remove the bacon and set it aside, reserving the bacon grease in the skillet.
2. Add the butter to the skillet and melt over medium heat. Add the garlic and sauté until fragrant, about 1 minute.
3. Pour in the white wine and lemon juice, and bring to a simmer.
4. Add the clams, cover the skillet, and cook for 5-7 minutes, or until the clams have opened.
5. If any clams don't open, throw them away.
6. Stir in the cooked bacon and fresh parsley, and season with sea salt and black pepper.
7. Serve the clams in their broth with a side of crusty carnivore bread if desired.

Number of servings: 4

Preparation time: 10 minutes

Cooking time: 15 minutes

Nutritional value per serving:
Calories: 300, Carbs: 2g, Fiber: 0g, Sugars: 0g, Protein: 24g, Saturated fat: 8g, Unsaturated fat: 10g

Difficulty rating: ★★☆☆☆

Tips for ingredient variations: Add a pinch of smoked paprika for a deeper flavor.

Side Dishes

Bacon-Wrapped Asparagus

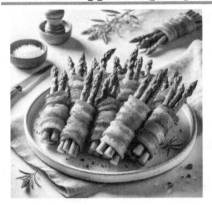

Ingredients:

- 1 lb asparagus spears, trimmed
- 12 slices bacon
- Sea salt and black pepper to taste

Directions:

1. Preheat your oven to 400°F (200°C).
2. Divide the asparagus into 12 bundles, with 3-4 spears per bundle.
3. Wrap each bundle tightly with a slice of bacon.
4. Place the bacon-wrapped asparagus bundles on a baking sheet lined with parchment paper.
5. Season with sea salt and black pepper.
6. Bake for 20 minutes, or until the bacon is crispy and the asparagus is tender.
7. Serve warm.

Number of servings: 4

Preparation time: 10 minutes

Cooking time: 20 minutes

Nutritional value per serving:
Calories: 200, Carbs: 4g, Fiber: 2g, Sugars: 2g, Protein: 10g, Saturated fat: 7g, Unsaturated fat: 5g

Difficulty rating: ★★☆☆☆

Tips for ingredient variations: Add a sprinkle of grated Parmesan cheese on top before baking for extra flavor.

Buttered Mushrooms

Number of servings: 4

Preparation time: 5 minutes

Cooking time: 10 minutes

Nutritional value per serving:
Calories: 100, Carbs: 4g, Fiber: 1g, Sugars: 1g, Protein: 2g, Saturated fat: 7g, Unsaturated fat: 1g

Difficulty rating: ★☆☆☆☆

Tips for ingredient variations: Use different varieties of mushrooms like cremini, shiitake, or portobello for a richer flavor profile.

Directions:

1. Melt the butter over medium heat in a large skillet.
2. Add the garlic and simmer for one minute, until fragrant.
3. Add the mushrooms and simmer for 8 to 10 minutes, stirring now and again, until they are soft and golden brown.
4. Season with sea salt and black pepper.
5. Garnish with chopped parsley if desired.
6. Serve warm.

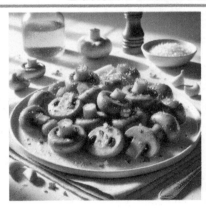

Ingredients:

- 1 lb mushrooms, cleaned and sliced
- 4 tablespoons butter
- 2 cloves garlic, minced
- Sea salt and black pepper to taste
- Fresh parsley, chopped (optional)

Cheesy Cauliflower Mash (Carnivore Style)

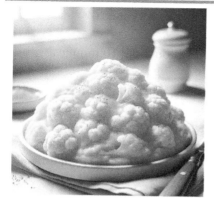

Ingredients:

• 1 large head of cauliflower, chopped into florets
• 4 tablespoons butter
• 1/2 cup heavy cream
• 1 cup shredded cheddar cheese
• Sea salt and black pepper to taste

Directions:

1. Steam the cauliflower florets until tender, about 10-12 minutes.
2. Drain well and transfer to a food processor.
3. Add the butter, heavy cream, and shredded cheddar cheese.
4. Blend until smooth and creamy.
5. Season with sea salt and black pepper to taste.
6. Serve warm.

Number of servings: 4

Preparation time: 10 minutes

Cooking time: 20 minutes

Nutritional value per serving:
Calories: 210, Carbs: 5g, Fiber: 2g, Sugars: 2g, Protein: 6g, Saturated fat: 14g, Unsaturated fat: 3g

Difficulty rating: ★★☆☆

Tips for ingredient variations: Add a clove of roasted garlic or a tablespoon of sour cream for additional flavor.

Roasted Bone Marrow

Number of servings: 4

Preparation time: 5 minutes

Cooking time: 25 minutes

Nutritional value per serving:
Calories: 180, Carbs: 0g, Fiber: 0g, Sugars: 0g, Protein: 4g, Saturated fat: 10g, Unsaturated fat: 7g

Difficulty rating: ★☆☆☆

Tips for ingredient variations:
Serve with a sprinkle of sea salt and freshly cracked black pepper for enhanced flavor.

Directions:

1. Preheat your oven to 450°F (230°C).
2. Place the marrow bones on a baking sheet lined with parchment paper.
3. Season with sea salt and black pepper.
4. Roast in the oven for 20-25 minutes, until the marrow is soft and bubbly.
5. Garnish with chopped parsley and serve with lemon wedges if desired.
6. Serve warm, scooping the marrow out of the bones.

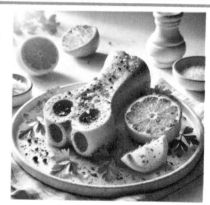

Ingredients:

• 4 large beef marrow bones
• Sea salt and black pepper to taste
• Fresh parsley, chopped (optional)
• Lemon wedges (optional)

Crispy Pork Belly Bites

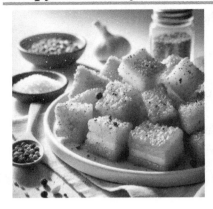

Ingredients:
- 1 lb pork belly, cut into bite-sized pieces
- Sea salt and black pepper to taste
- 1 teaspoon garlic powder
- 1 teaspoon onion powder
- 1 teaspoon smoked paprika

Directions:

1. Preheat your oven to 400°F (200°C).
2. Season the pork belly pieces with sea salt, black pepper, garlic powder, onion powder, and smoked paprika.
3. Place the seasoned pork belly pieces on a baking sheet lined with parchment paper.
4. Bake for 45-60 minutes, or until the pork belly is crispy and golden brown.
5. Serve warm.

Number of servings: 4

Preparation time: 10 minutes

Cooking time: 60 minutes

Nutritional value per serving:
Calories: 320, Carbs: 0g, Fiber: 0g, Sugars: 0g, Protein: 10g, Saturated fat: 14g, Unsaturated fat: 10g

Difficulty rating: ★★☆☆

Tips for ingredient variations: For an Asian twist, add a tablespoon of soy sauce or tamari to the seasoning mix.

Parmesan Crusted Zucchini Fries

Number of servings: 4
Preparation time: 15 minutes
Cooking time: 20 minutes
Nutritional value per serving:
Calories: 180, Carbs: 4g, Fiber: 2g, Sugars: 2g, Protein: 9g, Saturated fat: 4g, Unsaturated fat: 5g

Difficulty rating: ★★☆☆

Tips for ingredient variations: Add a sprinkle of red pepper flakes for a touch of heat, or serve with a side of marinara sauce for dipping.

Directions:

1. Preheat your oven to 425°F (220°C) and line a baking sheet with parchment paper.
2. Cut the zucchinis into fry-like strips, about 1/2 inch thick.
3. In a bowl, combine the Parmesan cheese, garlic powder, Italian seasoning, sea salt, and black pepper.
4. Toss the zucchini strips with olive oil, then coat them evenly with the Parmesan mixture.
5. Arrange the zucchini fries in a single layer on the prepared baking sheet.
6. Bake for 20 minutes or until golden and crispy, flipping halfway through.
7. Remove from the oven, garnish with fresh parsley if desired, and serve warm.

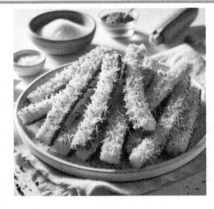

Ingredients:
- 4 medium zucchinis
- 1 cup grated Parmesan cheese
- 1 teaspoon garlic powder
- 1 teaspoon Italian seasoning
- Sea salt and black pepper to taste
- 2 tablespoons olive oil
- 1 tablespoon fresh parsley, chopped (optional)

Pan-Seared Scallops with Bacon

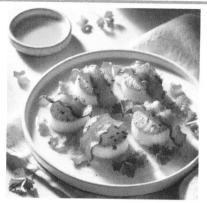

Ingredients:

- 12 large sea scallops
- 6 slices bacon, chopped
- 2 tablespoons butter
- Sea salt and black pepper to taste
- 1 tablespoon lemon juice
- Fresh parsley, chopped (optional)

Directions:

1. Cook the diced bacon in a big skillet over medium heat until it becomes crispy. Remove with a slotted spoon and set aside.
2. In the same skillet, melt the butter in the bacon fat.
3. Season the scallops with sea salt and black pepper.
4. Add the scallops to the skillet and cook for 2-3 minutes on each side until they develop a golden crust and are opaque in the center.
5. Remove from heat and stir in the lemon juice.
6. Top the scallops with the crispy bacon and garnish with fresh parsley if desired. Serve warm.

Number of servings: 4

Preparation time: 10 minutes

Cooking time: 10 minutes

Nutritional value per serving:
Calories: 250, Carbs: 1g, Fiber: 0g, Sugars: 0g, Protein: 20g, Saturated fat: 10g, Unsaturated fat: 7g

Difficulty rating: ★★☆☆

Tips for ingredient variations: For added flavor, deglaze the pan with a splash of white wine before adding the scallops.

Creamy Spinach (Carnivore Style)

Number of servings: 4

Preparation time: 10 minutes

Cooking time: 15 minutes

Nutritional value per serving:
Calories: 320, Carbs: 4g, Fiber: 2g, Sugars: 2g, Protein: 5g, Saturated fat: 28g, Unsaturated fat: 4g

Difficulty rating: ★★☆☆

Tips for ingredient variations: Add a pinch of nutmeg for a warm, spicy flavor.

Directions:

1. Heat a large skillet over medium heat to melt the butter.
2. After adding, sauté the minced garlic for one minute, or until fragrant.
3. Add the spinach to the skillet and cook until wilted, about 5 minutes.
4. Stir in the heavy cream and cream cheese, cooking until the mixture is smooth and creamy.
5. Season with sea salt and black pepper to taste.
6. Serve warm.

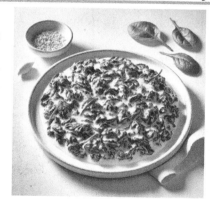

Ingredients:

- 1 lb fresh spinach, washed and chopped
- 1 cup heavy cream
- 1/2 cup cream cheese
- 4 tablespoons butter
- 2 cloves garlic, minced
- Sea salt and black pepper to taste

Bacon-Wrapped Jalapeños

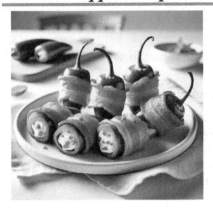

Ingredients:
• 8 large jalapeños, halved and seeded
• 4 ounces cream cheese, softened
• 8 slices bacon, halved

Directions:
1. Preheat your oven to 400°F (200°C). Line a baking sheet with parchment paper.
2. Fill each jalapeño half with a generous amount of cream cheese.
3. Wrap each filled jalapeño half with a slice of bacon and secure with a toothpick if needed.
4. Place the bacon-wrapped jalapeños on the prepared baking sheet.
5. Bake for 20-25 minutes, or until the bacon is crispy and the jalapeños are tender.
6. Allow to cool slightly before serving.

Number of servings: 4

Preparation time: 15 minutes

Cooking time: 25 minutes

Nutritional value per serving:
Calories: 250, Carbs: 2g, Fiber: 1g, Sugars: 1g, Protein: 9g, Saturated fat: 18g, Unsaturated fat: 5g

Difficulty rating: ★★☆☆☆

Tips for ingredient variations: For extra flavor, mix shredded cheddar cheese into the cream cheese before filling the jalapeños.

Carnivore Stuffed Peppers (Ground Meat and Cheese)

Number of servings: 4

Preparation time: 15 minutes

Cooking time: 35 minutes

Nutritional value per serving:
Calories: 400, Carbs: 6g, Fiber: 2g, Sugars: 3g, Protein: 30g, Saturated fat: 20g, Unsaturated fat: 10g

Difficulty rating: ★★☆☆☆

Tips for ingredient variations:
Use a mix of different cheeses for a richer flavor, such as mozzarella and Parmesan.

Directions:
1. Preheat your oven to 375°F (190°C).
2. Heat a large skillet over medium heat to melt the butter. Cook the minced garlic and diced onions until they become tender.
3. Cook until browned after adding the ground beef to the skillet. Season with sea salt and black pepper.
4. Remove from heat and stir in the shredded cheddar cheese.
5. Fill each bell pepper half with the meat and cheese mixture.
6. Place the stuffed peppers in a baking dish and bake for 30-35 minutes, or until the peppers are tender and the cheese is melted and bubbly.
7. Allow to cool slightly before serving.

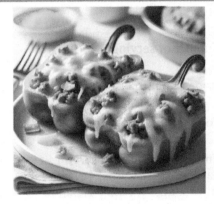

Ingredients:
• 4 large bell peppers, halved and seeded
• 1 lb ground beef
• 1 cup shredded cheddar cheese
• 1/2 cup diced onions
• 2 cloves garlic, minced
• 2 tablespoons butter
• Sea salt and black pepper to taste

Grilled Chicken Skewers

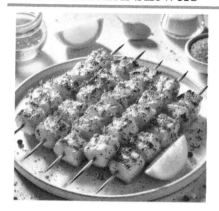

Ingredients:
• 1.5 pounds chicken breast, cut into 1-inch cubes
• 1/4 cup olive oil
• 2 tablespoons lemon juice
• 1 tablespoon dried oregano
• 1 teaspoon garlic powder
• Sea salt and black pepper to taste
• Wooden or metal skewers

Directions:
1. In a large bowl, combine the olive oil, lemon juice, oregano, garlic powder, sea salt, and black pepper. Mix well.
2. Add the chicken cubes to the bowl and toss to coat. Let marinate for at least 15 minutes.
3. Preheat the grill to medium-high heat.
4. Using skewers, thread the cubed chicken.
5. Grill the skewers for about 5 minutes on each side, or until the chicken is cooked through and has nice grill marks.
6. Serve warm.

Number of servings: 4

Preparation time: 20 minutes

Cooking time: 10 minutes

Nutritional value per serving:
Calories: 250, Carbs: 1g, Fiber: 0g, Sugars: 0g, Protein: 35g, Saturated fat: 3g, Unsaturated fat: 7g

Difficulty rating: ★★☆☆☆

Tips for ingredient variations: Add chunks of bell peppers and onions to the skewers for added flavor and texture.

Beef Tallow Roasted Brussels Sprouts

Number of servings: 4

Preparation time: 10 minutes

Cooking time: 30 minutes

Nutritional value per serving:
Calories: 150, Carbs: 7g, Fiber: 3g, Sugars: 2g, Protein: 3g, Saturated fat: 4g, Unsaturated fat: 2g

Difficulty rating: ★☆☆☆☆

Tips for ingredient variations: Add a squeeze of fresh lemon juice over the Brussels sprouts before serving for a burst of freshness.

Directions:
1. Preheat your oven to 400°F (200°C).
2. In a large bowl, toss the Brussels sprouts with melted beef tallow, sea salt, black pepper, garlic powder, and onion powder.
3. Spread the Brussels sprouts in a single layer on a baking sheet.
4. Roast for 25-30 minutes, or until the Brussels sprouts are crispy on the outside and tender on the inside, stirring halfway through.
5. Serve warm.

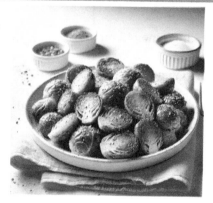

Ingredients:
• 1 pound Brussels sprouts, trimmed and halved
• 1/4 cup beef tallow, melted
• Sea salt and black pepper to taste
• 1 teaspoon garlic powder
• 1 teaspoon onion powder

Pork Rind Crusted Onion Rings

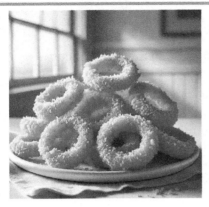

Ingredients:
- 2 large onions, sliced into rings
- 2 cups crushed pork rinds
- 1/2 cup grated Parmesan cheese
- 2 large eggs, beaten
- Sea salt and black pepper to taste

Directions:
1. Preheat your oven to 425°F (220°C). Line a baking sheet with parchment paper.
2. In a medium bowl, combine the crushed pork rinds, grated Parmesan cheese, sea salt, and black pepper.
3. Dip each onion ring into the beaten eggs, then coat with the pork rind mixture.
4. Place the coated onion rings on the prepared baking sheet.
5. Bake for 15 minutes, or until golden brown and crispy.
6. Serve warm.

Number of servings: 4

Preparation time: 15 minutes

Cooking time: 15 minutes

Nutritional value per serving:
Calories: 180, Carbs: 6g, Fiber: 1g, Sugars: 2g, Protein: 9g, Saturated fat: 4g, Unsaturated fat: 2g

Difficulty rating: ★★☆☆☆

Tips for ingredient variations: Add a pinch of cayenne pepper to the pork rind mixture for a spicy kick.

Herb Butter Roasted Chicken Wings

Number of servings: 4

Preparation time: 10 minutes

Cooking time: 45 minutes

Nutritional value per serving:
Calories: 320, Carbs: 0g, Fiber: 0g, Sugars: 0g, Protein: 25g, Saturated fat: 10g, Unsaturated fat: 12g

Difficulty rating: ★★☆☆☆

Tips for ingredient variations: Add a squeeze of fresh lemon juice over the wings before serving for added zest.

Directions:
1. Preheat your oven to 400°F (200°C). Line a baking sheet with parchment paper.
2. In a large bowl, combine the melted butter, rosemary, thyme, garlic powder, sea salt, and black pepper.
3. Add the chicken wings to the bowl and toss to coat.
4. Arrange the chicken wings in a single layer on the prepared baking sheet.
5. Roast for 40-45 minutes, or until the wings are golden brown and crispy, turning halfway through.
6. Serve warm.

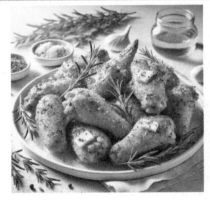

Ingredients:
- 2 pounds chicken wings
- 1/4 cup butter, melted
- 2 tablespoons fresh rosemary, chopped
- 2 tablespoons fresh thyme, chopped
- 1 teaspoon garlic powder
- Sea salt and black pepper to taste

Sausage and Cheese Stuffed Mushrooms

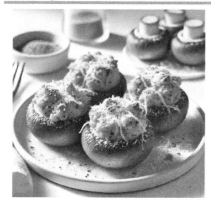

Ingredients:
- 12 large button mushrooms, stems removed
- 1/2 pound ground sausage
- 1/2 cup cream cheese, softened
- 1/4 cup grated Parmesan cheese
- 1/4 teaspoon garlic powder
- Sea salt and black pepper to taste

Directions:
1. Preheat your oven to 375°F (190°C). Line a baking sheet with parchment paper.
2. Cook the ground sausage in a pan over medium heat until it is well browned. Remove from heat and drain any excess fat.
3. In a medium bowl, combine the cooked sausage, cream cheese, grated Parmesan cheese, garlic powder, sea salt, and black pepper.
4. Stuff each mushroom cap with the sausage mixture and place on the prepared baking sheet.
5. Bake for 20 to 25 minutes, until the filling is golden brown and the mushrooms are soft.
6. Serve warm.

Number of servings: 4

Preparation time: 20 minutes

Cooking time: 25 minutes

Nutritional value per serving:
Calories: 210, Carbs: 4g, Fiber: 1g, Sugars: 2g, Protein: 12g, Saturated fat: 10g, Unsaturated fat: 4g

Difficulty rating: ★★☆☆☆

Tips for ingredient variations:
Add chopped fresh parsley to the sausage mixture for a burst of color and flavor.

Desserts

Carnivore Cheesecake (Cream Cheese and Eggs)

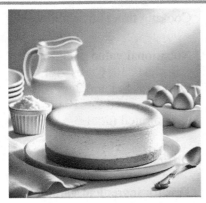

Ingredients:
- 16 ounces cream cheese, softened
- 3 large eggs
- 1 cup sour cream
- ½ cup heavy cream
- 1 teaspoon vanilla extract
- ½ cup erythritol (optional, for sweetness)
- Pinch of sea salt

Directions:
1. Preheat your oven to 325°F (165°C).
2. In a large bowl, beat the cream cheese until smooth.
3. Beat thoroughly after each addition of egg. Add the eggs one at a time.
4. Mix in the sour cream, heavy cream, vanilla extract, erythritol (if using), and sea salt until fully combined.
5. Pour the mixture into a greased 9-inch springform pan.
6. Bake for 50 to 60 minutes, until the top is lightly brown and the middle is set.
7. Allow the cheesecake to cool to room temperature, then refrigerate for at least 4 hours before serving.

Number of servings: 8

Preparation time: 15 minutes

Cooking time: 1 hour

Nutritional value per serving: Calories: 350, Carbs: 2g, Fiber: 0g, Sugars: 1g, Protein: 6g, Saturated fat: 30g, Unsaturated fat: 10g

Difficulty rating: ★★☆☆☆

Tips for ingredient variations: Add a teaspoon of lemon zest for a refreshing twist.

Egg Custard

Number of servings: 6

Preparation time: 10 minutes

Cooking time: 30 minutes

Nutritional value per serving: Calories: 250, Carbs: 2g, Fiber: 0g, Sugars: 1g, Protein: 6g, Saturated fat: 20g, Unsaturated fat: 5g

Difficulty rating: ★★☆☆☆

Tips for ingredient variations: Add a dash of cinnamon for additional warmth and flavor.

Directions:
1. Preheat your oven to 350°F (175°C).
2. In a large bowl, whisk together the eggs, heavy cream, vanilla extract, erythritol (if using), and sea salt until well combined.
3. Pour the mixture into six individual ramekins.
4. After setting the ramekins in a baking dish, cover the sides with hot water halfway up.
5. Bake the custards for 30 minutes, or until they are set but the center is still a little wobbly.
6. Remove from the oven and let cool. Sprinkle with ground nutmeg before serving.

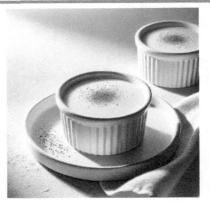

Ingredients:
- 4 large eggs
- 2 cups heavy cream
- 1 teaspoon vanilla extract
- ¼ cup erythritol (optional, for sweetness)
- Pinch of sea salt
- Ground nutmeg, for garnish

Cream Cheese Clouds

Ingredients:
- 8 ounces cream cheese, softened
- 2 large eggs
- 2 tablespoons butter, melted
- 1 teaspoon vanilla extract
- ¼ cup erythritol (optional, for sweetness)
- Pinch of sea salt

Directions:
1. Preheat your oven to 350°F (175°C) and line a baking sheet with parchment paper.
2. In a large bowl, beat the cream cheese until smooth.
3. Add the eggs, melted butter, vanilla extract, erythritol (if using), and sea salt. Mix until well combined.
4. Drop spoonfuls of the mixture onto the prepared baking sheet, spacing them about 2 inches apart.
5. Bake for 12-15 minutes, or until the edges are golden brown.
6. After a few minutes of cooling on the baking sheet, move the clouds to a wire rack to finish cooling.

Number of servings: 12
Preparation time: 10 minutes
Cooking time: 15 minutes
Nutritional value per serving: Calories: 110, Carbs: 1g, Fiber: 0g, Sugars: 0g, Protein: 3g, Saturated fat: 10g, Unsaturated fat: 3g

Difficulty rating: ★☆☆☆☆
Tips for ingredient variations: Add a few drops of lemon or almond extract for a different flavor profile.

Carnivore Ice Cream (Eggs and Heavy Cream)

Number of servings: 6
Preparation time: 10 minutes (plus freezing time)
Cooking time: 10 minutes
Nutritional value per serving: Calories: 300, Carbs: 2g, Fiber: 0g, Sugars: 1g, Protein: 3g, Saturated fat: 28g, Unsaturated fat: 8g

Difficulty rating: ★★☆☆☆
Tips for ingredient variations: Swirl in some melted dark chocolate for a chocolate marble effect.

Directions:
1. In a medium saucepan, whisk together the egg yolks, heavy cream, vanilla extract, erythritol (if using), and sea salt.
2. Cook over medium heat, stirring constantly, until the mixture thickens enough to coat the back of a spoon.
3. Remove from heat and let cool to room temperature.
4. Pour the mixture into an ice cream maker and churn according to the manufacturer's instructions.
5. Transfer to a container and freeze for at least 2 hours before serving.

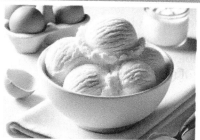

Ingredients:
- 4 large egg yolks
- 2 cups heavy cream
- 1 teaspoon vanilla extract
- ¼ cup erythritol (optional, for sweetness)
- Pinch of sea salt

Beef Tallow Chocolate Fudge

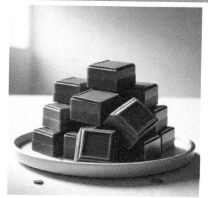

Ingredients:
- 1 cup beef tallow
- ½ cup cocoa powder
- ¼ cup erythritol (optional, for sweetness)
- 1 teaspoon vanilla extract
- Pinch of sea salt

Directions:
1. In a medium saucepan, melt the beef tallow over low heat.
2. Remove from heat and whisk in the cocoa powder, erythritol (if using), vanilla extract, and sea salt until smooth.
3. Pour the mixture into a lined 8x8 inch baking dish.
4. Refrigerate for at least 2 hours, or until the fudge is set.
5. Cut into 16 squares and serve chilled.

Number of servings: 16
Preparation time: 10 minutes
Cooking time: 5 minutes (plus chilling time)
Nutritional value per serving: Calories: 120, Carbs: 1g, Fiber: 0g, Sugars: 0g, Protein: 1g, Saturated fat: 10g, Unsaturated fat: 2g

Difficulty rating: ★☆☆☆☆
Tips for ingredient variations: Add a tablespoon of instant coffee granules to enhance the chocolate flavor.

Whipped Cream with Gelatin

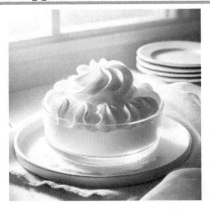

Ingredients:
• 1 cup heavy cream
• 1 tablespoon gelatin
• 1 tablespoon cold water
• 1 teaspoon vanilla extract
• 1-2 tablespoons powdered erythritol (optional)

Directions:
1. Allow the gelatin to bloom for five minutes after sprinkling it over the cold water in a small bowl.
2. Heat the bloomed gelatin in the microwave for 10-15 seconds until melted.
3. In a large bowl, whip the heavy cream until soft peaks form.
4. Add the melted gelatin, vanilla extract, and powdered erythritol (if using) to the whipped cream.
5. Continue whipping until stiff peaks form.
6. Serve immediately or refrigerate for up to 24 hours.

Number of servings: 4

Preparation time: 10 minutes

Cooking time: 5 minutes

Nutritional value per serving:
Calories: 210, Carbs: 1g, Fiber: 0g, Sugars: 0g, Protein: 3g, Saturated fat: 14g, Unsaturated fat: 5g

Difficulty rating: ★★☆☆

Tips for ingredient variations: Add 1 teaspoon of cocoa powder for a chocolate-flavored whipped cream.

Pork Rind Cookies

Number of servings: 12 cookies

Preparation time: 10 minutes

Cooking time: 15 minutes

Nutritional value per serving:
Calories: 150, Carbs: 2g, Fiber: 1g, Sugars: 0g, Protein: 5g, Saturated fat: 6g, Unsaturated fat: 4g

Difficulty rating: ★★☆☆

Tips for ingredient variations: Add 1/4 cup sugar-free chocolate chips to the dough for a chocolatey twist.

Directions:
1. Preheat your oven to 350°F (175°C) and line a baking sheet with parchment paper.
2. In a large bowl, mix together the crushed pork rinds, almond flour, melted butter, powdered erythritol, vanilla extract, and egg until well combined.
3. Using the back of the spoon, gently flatten each cookie as you drop spoonfuls of dough onto the baking sheet that has been prepared.
4. Bake for 12-15 minutes, or until the edges are golden brown.
5. After five minutes of cooling on the baking sheet, move the cookies to a wire rack to finish cooling.

Ingredients:
• 1 cup crushed pork rinds
• 1 cup almond flour
• 1/2 cup melted butter
• 1/4 cup powdered erythritol
• 1 teaspoon vanilla extract
• 1 large egg

Butter Mousse

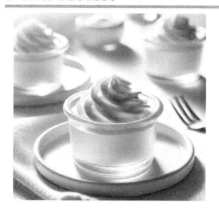

Ingredients:

- 1 cup unsalted butter, softened
- 1/4 cup powdered erythritol
- 1 teaspoon vanilla extract
- 1/2 cup heavy cream

Directions:

1. In a large bowl, beat the softened butter with the powdered erythritol and vanilla extract until light and fluffy.
2. Beat the heavy cream in a separate dish until firm peaks form.
3. Gently fold the whipped cream into the butter mixture until well combined.
4. Spoon the mousse into serving dishes and refrigerate for at least 1 hour before serving.

Number of servings: 4

Preparation time: 10 minutes

Cooking time: 0 minutes

Nutritional value per serving:
Calories: 320, Carbs: 1g, Fiber: 0g, Sugars: 0g, Protein: 1g, Saturated fat: 30g, Unsaturated fat: 4g

Difficulty rating: ★★☆☆

Tips for ingredient variations: Add a pinch of sea salt for a salted butter mousse.

Vanilla Egg Pudding

Number of servings: 4

Preparation time: 10 minutes

Cooking time: 15 minutes

Nutritional value per serving:
Calories: 300, Carbs: 3g, Fiber: 0g, Sugars: 2g, Protein: 5g, Saturated fat: 25g, Unsaturated fat: 5g

Difficulty rating: ★★☆☆

Tips for ingredient variations: Add a pinch of ground cinnamon for a spiced vanilla egg pudding.

Directions:

1. In a medium saucepan, whisk together the eggs, heavy cream, and powdered erythritol.
2. Stirring frequently, cook over medium heat until the mixture thickens and coats the back of a spoon, about 10 to 15 minutes.
3. Remove from heat and stir in the vanilla extract.
4. Pour the pudding into individual serving dishes and refrigerate for at least 2 hours before serving.

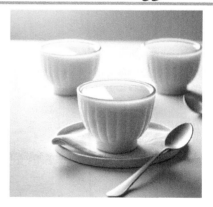

Ingredients:

- 4 large eggs
- 2 cups heavy cream
- 1/4 cup powdered erythritol
- 1 teaspoon vanilla extract

Bone Marrow Custard

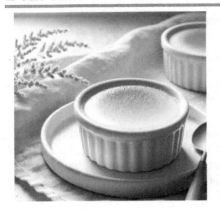

Ingredients:

- 1/2 cup bone marrow, softened
- 2 cups heavy cream
- 4 large egg yolks
- 1/4 cup powdered erythritol
- 1 teaspoon vanilla extract

Directions:

1. Preheat your oven to 325°F (165°C).
2. In a blender, combine the softened bone marrow, heavy cream, egg yolks, powdered erythritol, and vanilla extract. Blend until smooth.
3. Pour the mixture into ramekins or custard cups.
4. Fill the baking dish halfway up the sides of the ramekins with hot water after placing the ramekins inside.
5. Bake for 40 to 45 minutes, or until the custard is set through but the middle is still a little jiggly.
6. After taking the ramekins out of the water bath, allow them to reach room temperature. Refrigerate for at least 2 hours before serving.

Number of servings: 4

Preparation time: 15 minutes

Cooking time: 45 minutes

Nutritional value per serving: Calories: 320, Carbs: 2g, Fiber: 0g, Sugars: 0g, Protein: 5g, Saturated fat: 25g, Unsaturated fat: 5g

Difficulty rating: ★★★☆☆

Tips for ingredient variations: Top with a sprinkle of sea salt for a savory twist.

Coconut Oil Chocolate Bars

Number of servings: 10

Preparation time: 10 minutes

Cooking time: 30 minutes (chilling time)

Nutritional value per serving: Calories: 210, Carbs: 3g, Fiber: 1g, Sugars: 0g, Protein: 1g, Saturated fat: 20g, Unsaturated fat: 2g

Difficulty rating: ★☆☆☆☆

Tips for ingredient variations: Add 1/4 cup of crushed nuts for added texture and flavor.

Directions:

1. In a medium bowl, mix together the melted coconut oil, cocoa powder, powdered erythritol, vanilla extract, and sea salt until smooth and well combined.
2. Transfer the blend into a baking dish coated with parchment paper or a silicone mold.
3. Place in the refrigerator and chill for at least 30 minutes, or until set.
4. Once set, remove from the mold or baking dish and cut into bars.

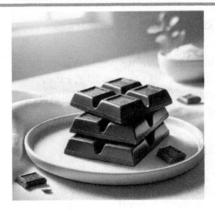

Ingredients:

- 1 cup coconut oil, melted
- 1/2 cup unsweetened cocoa powder
- 1/4 cup powdered erythritol (optional, for sweetness)
- 1 teaspoon vanilla extract
- Pinch of sea salt

Lemon Ricotta Cake

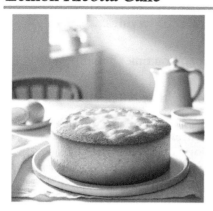

Ingredients:

- 1 1/2 cups ricotta cheese
- 3 large eggs
- 1/2 cup coconut flour
- 1/4 cup lemon juice
- 1 tablespoon lemon zest
- 1/4 cup powdered erythritol (optional, for sweetness)
- 1 teaspoon vanilla extract
- 1 teaspoon baking powder
- Pinch of sea salt

Directions:

1. Preheat your oven to 350°F (175°C). Grease an 8-inch round cake pan and line the bottom with parchment paper.
2. In a large bowl, whisk together the ricotta cheese, eggs, lemon juice, lemon zest, powdered erythritol, and vanilla extract until smooth.
3. In a separate bowl, mix the coconut flour, baking powder, and sea salt.
4. Combine the dry ingredients with the wet ingredients and mix until well combined.
5. Using a spatula, level the top of the batter after pouring it into the prepared cake pan.
6. Bake for forty-five minutes, or until a toothpick inserted in the center comes out clean.
7. Allow the cake to cool in the pan for 10 minutes, then transfer to a wire rack to cool completely.

Number of servings: 8

Preparation time: 15 minutes

Cooking time: 45 minutes

Nutritional value per serving: Calories: 190, Carbs: 5g, Fiber: 2g, Sugars: 2g, Protein: 8g, Saturated fat: 5g, Unsaturated fat: 2g

Difficulty rating: ★★★☆☆

Tips for ingredient variations: For a richer flavor, add 1/4 cup of heavy cream to the batter.

Salted Caramel Fat Bombs

Number of servings: 12

Preparation time: 10 minutes

Cooking time: 30 minutes (chilling time)

Nutritional value per serving: Calories: 150, Carbs: 2g, Fiber: 1g, Sugars: 0g, Protein: 1g, Saturated fat: 12g, Unsaturated fat: 3g

Difficulty rating: ★☆☆☆☆

Tips for ingredient variations: Add a sprinkle of coarse sea salt on top before chilling for an extra salty kick.

Directions:

1. In a medium saucepan, melt the butter, coconut oil, and almond butter over low heat, stirring until smooth.
2. Remove from heat and stir in the powdered erythritol, vanilla extract, and sea salt until well combined.
3. Transfer the blend into a baking dish coated with parchment paper or a silicone mold.
4. Place in the refrigerator and chill for at least 30 minutes, or until set.
5. Once set, remove from the mold or baking dish and cut into bite-sized pieces.

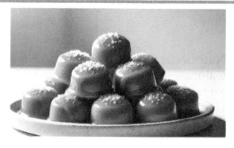

Ingredients:

- 1/2 cup butter
- 1/2 cup coconut oil
- 1/4 cup almond butter
- 1/4 cup powdered erythritol (optional, for sweetness)
- 1 teaspoon vanilla extract
- 1/2 teaspoon sea salt

Cream Cheese Pancakes

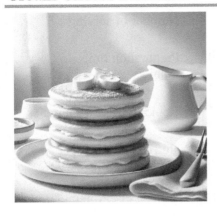

Ingredients:
- 2 large eggs
- 2 ounces cream cheese, softened
- 1/2 teaspoon cinnamon (optional)
- 1/2 teaspoon vanilla extract
- Butter, for cooking

Directions:
1. In a blender, combine the eggs, cream cheese, cinnamon, and vanilla extract. Blend until smooth.
2. Add a tiny bit of butter to a nonstick skillet and heat it over medium heat.
3. Pour the batter onto the skillet to form small pancakes. Fry until surface bubbles appear, then turn and continue cooking until both sides are golden brown.
4. Serve warm with additional butter if desired.

Number of servings: 2

Preparation time: 5 minutes

Cooking time: 10 minutes

Nutritional value per serving:
Calories: 200, Carbs: 2g, Fiber: 0g, Sugars: 1g, Protein: 8g, Saturated fat: 16g, Unsaturated fat: 3g

Difficulty rating: ★★☆☆☆

Tips for ingredient variations: Add a tablespoon of almond flour for a slightly thicker texture.

Bacon and Maple Fat Bombs

Number of servings: 12

Preparation time: 15 minutes

Cooking time: 30 minutes (chilling time)

Nutritional value per serving:
Calories: 160, Carbs: 1g, Fiber: 0g, Sugars: 0g, Protein: 3g, Saturated fat: 14g, Unsaturated fat: 2g

Difficulty rating: ★★☆☆☆

Tips for ingredient variations: Add 1/4 teaspoon of vanilla extract for an added flavor dimension.

Directions:
1. In a medium bowl, mix together the softened butter, cream cheese, melted coconut oil, and sugar-free maple syrup until smooth.
2. Fold in the crumbled bacon.
3. Transfer the blend into a silicone mold or a baking dish lined with parchment paper.
4. Place in the refrigerator and chill for at least 30 minutes, or until set.
5. Once set, remove from the mold or baking dish and cut into bite-sized pieces.

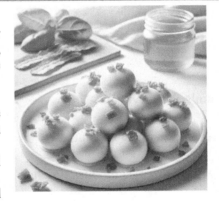

Ingredients:
- 1/2 cup butter, softened
- 1/2 cup cream cheese, softened
- 1/4 cup coconut oil, melted
- 2 tablespoons sugar-free maple syrup
- 6 slices bacon, cooked and crumbled

60-Day Carnivore Diet Meal Plan

Week 1:

Day 1

- Breakfast: Egg & Ham Bake
- Starter: Beef Tartare
- Main Dish: Ribeye Steak with Garlic Butter
- Side Dish: Bacon-Wrapped Asparagus
- Dessert: Carnivore Cheesecake (Cream Cheese and Eggs)

Day 2

- Breakfast: Bacon & Cheddar Breakfast Muffins
- Starter: Deviled Eggs with Bacon Bits
- Main Dish: Slow Cooker Beef Brisket
- Side Dish: Buttered Mushrooms
- Dessert: Egg Custard

Day 3

- Breakfast: Sausage & Cheese Breakfast Casserole
- Starter: Chicken Liver Pâté
- Main Dish: Grilled Lamb Chops
- Side Dish: Cheesy Cauliflower Mash (Carnivore Style)
- Dessert: Cream Cheese Clouds

Day 4

- Breakfast: Poached Eggs
- Starter: Pork Rind Nachos
- Main Dish: Beef Tenderloin with Blue Cheese Crust
- Side Dish: Roasted Bone Marrow
- Dessert: Carnivore Ice Cream (Eggs and Heavy Cream)

Day 5

- Breakfast: Scrambled Eggs with Butter
- Starter: Cheese-Stuffed Mushrooms (Carnivore Version)
- Main Dish: Smoked Beef Ribs
- Side Dish: Crispy Pork Belly Bites
- Dessert: Beef Tallow Chocolate Fudge

Day 6

- Breakfast: Omelet with Cheddar Cheese
- Starter: Beef Carpaccio
- Main Dish: Ground Beef Carnivore Chili
- Side Dish: Parmesan Crusted Zucchini Fries
- Dessert: Whipped Cream with Gelatin

Day 7

- Breakfast: Soft-Boiled Eggs with Sea Salt
- Starter: Bone Marrow Butter on Toasted Carnivore Bread
- Main Dish: Beef and Lamb Meatloaf
- Side Dish: Pan-Seared Scallops with Bacon
- Dessert: Pork Rind Cookies

Week 2:

Day 8

- Breakfast: Egg Muffins with Sausage
- Starter: Prosciutto-Wrapped Asparagus
- Main Dish: Braised Short Ribs
- Side Dish: Creamy Spinach (Carnivore Style)
- Dessert: Butter Mousse

Day 9

- Breakfast: Carnivore Pancakes (Egg and Pork Rinds)
- Starter: Crispy Chicken Skins
- Main Dish: Grilled T-Bone Steak
- Side Dish: Bacon-Wrapped Jalapeños
- Dessert: Vanilla Egg Pudding

Day 10

- Breakfast: Steak and Eggs
- Starter: Lamb Meatballs with Mint Sauce
- Main Dish: Chuck Roast with Bone Broth Gravy
- Side Dish: Carnivore Stuffed Peppers (Ground Meat and Cheese)
- Dessert: Bone Marrow Custard

Day 11

- Breakfast: Eggs Benedict with Hollandaise Sauce

- Starter: Shrimp Cocktail (with Carnivore Sauce)
- Main Dish: Beef and Liver Burgers
- Side Dish: Grilled Chicken Skewers
- Dessert: Coconut Oil Chocolate Bars

Day 12
- Breakfast: Carnivore Breakfast Pizza (Eggs, Bacon, Cheese)
- Starter: Carnivore Charcuterie Board
- Main Dish: Spicy Beef Tongue Tacos (Carnivore Style)
- Side Dish: Beef Tallow Roasted Brussels Sprouts
- Dessert: Lemon Ricotta Cake

Week 3:

Day 15
- Breakfast: Smoked Salmon and Scrambled Eggs
- Starter: Carnivore Sushi (Beef and Tuna)
- Main Dish: Beef Shank Osso Buco
- Side Dish: Sausage and Cheese Stuffed Mushrooms
- Dessert: Bacon and Maple Fat Bombs

Day 16
- Breakfast: Chicken Liver and Eggs
- Starter: Bacon-Wrapped Jalapeño Poppers
- Main Dish: Veal Cutlets with Lemon Butter Sauce
- Side Dish: Bacon-Wrapped Asparagus
- Dessert: Carnivore Cheesecake (Cream Cheese and Eggs)

Day 17
- Breakfast: Lamb Kidney and Egg Scramble
- Starter: Salmon Caviar on Egg Slices
- Main Dish: Lamb Shoulder Roast
- Side Dish: Buttered Mushrooms
- Dessert: Egg Custard

Day 18
- Breakfast: Duck Egg Omelet
- Starter: Bacon-Wrapped Scallops

Week 4:

Day 22
- Breakfast: Scrambled Eggs with Butter
- Starter: Pork Rind Nachos
- Main Dish: Bacon-Wrapped Chicken Breasts
- Side Dish: Pan-Seared Scallops with Bacon
- Dessert: Pork Rind Cookies

Day 13
- Breakfast: Meat Lover's Breakfast Skillet (Bacon, Sausage, Eggs)
- Starter: Grilled Octopus Tentacles
- Main Dish: Venison Stew
- Side Dish: Pork Rind Crusted Onion Rings
- Dessert: Salted Caramel Fat Bombs

Day 14
- Breakfast: Bone Broth Breakfast Soup
- Starter: Duck Liver Mousse
- Main Dish: Garlic Herb Prime Rib
- Side Dish: Herb Butter Roasted Chicken Wings
- Dessert: Cream Cheese Pancakes

- Main Dish: Bison Ribeye with Horseradish Cream
- Side Dish: Cheesy Cauliflower Mash (Carnivore Style)
- Dessert: Cream Cheese Clouds

Day 19
- Breakfast: Beef Liver and Onion Omelet
- Starter: Beef Tartare
- Main Dish: Roast Chicken with Herb Butter
- Side Dish: Roasted Bone Marrow
- Dessert: Carnivore Ice Cream (Eggs and Heavy Cream)

Day 20
- Breakfast: Cream Cheese and Egg Puffs
- Starter: Deviled Eggs with Bacon Bits
- Main Dish: Duck Breast with Crispy Skin
- Side Dish: Crispy Pork Belly Bites
- Dessert: Beef Tallow Chocolate Fudge

Day 21
- Breakfast: Poached Eggs
- Starter: Chicken Liver Pâté
- Main Dish: Chicken Thighs in Cream Sauce
- Side Dish: Parmesan Crusted Zucchini Fries
- Dessert: Whipped Cream with Gelatin

Day 23
- Breakfast: Omelet with Cheddar Cheese
- Starter: Cheese-Stuffed Mushrooms (Carnivore Version)
- Main Dish: Turkey Drumsticks with Garlic Butter
- Side Dish: Creamy Spinach (Carnivore Style)

- Dessert: Butter Mousse

Day 24

- Breakfast: Soft-Boiled Eggs with Sea Salt
- Starter: Beef Carpaccio
- Main Dish: Grilled Chicken Wings
- Side Dish: Bacon-Wrapped Jalapeños
- Dessert: Vanilla Egg Pudding

Day 25

- Breakfast: Egg Muffins with Sausage
- Starter: Bone Marrow Butter on Toasted Carnivore Bread
- Main Dish: Rabbit Stew
- Side Dish: Carnivore Stuffed Peppers (Ground Meat and Cheese)
- Dessert: Bone Marrow Custard

Day 26

- Breakfast: Carnivore Pancakes (Egg and Pork Rinds)
- Starter: Prosciutto-Wrapped Asparagus

Week 5:

Day 29

- Breakfast: Carnivore Breakfast Pizza (Eggs, Bacon, Cheese)
- Starter: Shrimp Cocktail (with Carnivore Sauce)
- Main Dish: Goose Breast with Red Wine Reduction
- Side Dish: Herb Butter Roasted Chicken Wings
- Dessert: Cream Cheese Pancakes

Day 30

- Breakfast: Meat Lover's Breakfast Skillet (Bacon, Sausage, Eggs)
- Starter: Carnivore Charcuterie Board
- Main Dish: Lemon Garlic Chicken Skewers
- Side Dish: Sausage and Cheese Stuffed Mushrooms
- Dessert: Bacon and Maple Fat Bombs

Day 31

- Breakfast: Bone Broth Breakfast Soup
- Starter: Grilled Octopus Tentacles
- Main Dish: Pork Tenderloin with Apple Reduction
- Side Dish: Bacon-Wrapped Asparagus
- Dessert: Carnivore Cheesecake (Cream Cheese and Eggs)

- Main Dish: Pheasant Breast with Mustard Sauce
- Side Dish: Grilled Chicken Skewers
- Dessert: Coconut Oil Chocolate Bars

Day 27

- Breakfast: Steak and Eggs
- Starter: Crispy Chicken Skins
- Main Dish: Slow-Cooked Duck Legs
- Side Dish: Beef Tallow Roasted Brussels Sprouts
- Dessert: Lemon Ricotta Cake

Day 28

- Breakfast: Eggs Benedict with Hollandaise Sauce
- Starter: Lamb Meatballs with Mint Sauce
- Main Dish: Chicken Alfredo (Carnivore Style)
- Side Dish: Pork Rind Crusted Onion Rings
- Dessert: Salted Caramel Fat Bombs

Day 32

- Breakfast: Smoked Salmon and Scrambled Eggs
- Starter: Duck Liver Mousse
- Main Dish: Stuffed Turkey Thighs
- Side Dish: Buttered Mushrooms
- Dessert: Egg Custard

Day 33

- Breakfast: Chicken Liver and Eggs
- Starter: Carnivore Sushi (Beef and Tuna)
- Main Dish: Chicken Liver Stroganoff
- Side Dish: Cheesy Cauliflower Mash (Carnivore Style)
- Dessert: Cream Cheese Clouds

Day 34

- Breakfast: Lamb Kidney and Egg Scramble
- Starter: Bacon-Wrapped Jalapeño Poppers
- Main Dish: BBQ Chicken Drumsticks
- Side Dish: Roasted Bone Marrow
- Dessert: Carnivore Ice Cream (Eggs and Heavy Cream)

Day 35

- Breakfast: Duck Egg Omelet
- Starter: Salmon Caviar on Egg Slices
- Main Dish: Pan-Seared Quail
- Side Dish: Crispy Pork Belly Bites
- Dessert: Beef Tallow Chocolate Fudge

Week 6:

Day 36
- Breakfast: Beef Liver and Onion Omelet
- Starter: Bacon-Wrapped Scallops
- Main Dish: Rabbit Sausage Patties
- Side Dish: Parmesan Crusted Zucchini Fries
- Dessert: Whipped Cream with Gelatin

Day 37
- Breakfast: Cream Cheese and Egg Puffs
- Starter: Beef Tartare
- Main Dish: Butter-Basted Lobster Tails
- Side Dish: Pan-Seared Scallops with Bacon
- Dessert: Pork Rind Cookies

Day 38
- Breakfast: Poached Eggs
- Starter: Deviled Eggs with Bacon Bits
- Main Dish: Garlic Shrimp Scampi
- Side Dish: Creamy Spinach (Carnivore Style)
- Dessert: Butter Mousse

Day 39
- Breakfast: Scrambled Eggs with Butter
- Starter: Chicken Liver Pâté
- Main Dish: Pan-Seared Scallops with Lemon Butter

Week 7:

Day 43
- Breakfast: Carnivore Pancakes (Egg and Pork Rinds)
- Starter: Bone Marrow Butter on Toasted Carnivore Bread
- Main Dish: Broiled Oysters with Herb Butter
- Side Dish: Pork Rind Crusted Onion Rings
- Dessert: Salted Caramel Fat Bombs

Day 44
- Breakfast: Steak and Eggs
- Starter: Prosciutto-Wrapped Asparagus
- Main Dish: Smoked Mackerel
- Side Dish: Herb Butter Roasted Chicken Wings
- Dessert: Cream Cheese Pancakes

Day 45
- Breakfast: Eggs Benedict with Hollandaise Sauce
- Starter: Crispy Chicken Skins
- Main Dish: Tuna Steaks with Wasabi Butter
- Side Dish: Sausage and Cheese Stuffed Mushrooms

- Side Dish: Bacon-Wrapped Jalapeños
- Dessert: Vanilla Egg Pudding

Day 40
- Breakfast: Omelet with Cheddar Cheese
- Starter: Pork Rind Nachos
- Main Dish: Grilled Swordfish Steaks
- Side Dish: Carnivore Stuffed Peppers (Ground Meat and Cheese)
- Dessert: Bone Marrow Custard

Day 41
- Breakfast: Soft-Boiled Eggs with Sea Salt
- Starter: Cheese-Stuffed Mushrooms (Carnivore Version)
- Main Dish: Salmon Fillet with Dill Sauce
- Side Dish: Grilled Chicken Skewers
- Dessert: Coconut Oil Chocolate Bars

Day 42
- Breakfast: Egg Muffins with Sausage
- Starter: Beef Carpaccio
- Main Dish: Crab Cakes (Carnivore Style)
- Side Dish: Beef Tallow Roasted Brussels Sprouts
- Dessert: Lemon Ricotta Cake

- Dessert: Bacon and Maple Fat Bombs

Day 46
- Breakfast: Carnivore Breakfast Pizza (Eggs, Bacon, Cheese)
- Starter: Lamb Meatballs with Mint Sauce
- Main Dish: Grilled Octopus with Olive Oil
- Side Dish: Bacon-Wrapped Asparagus
- Dessert: Carnivore Cheesecake (Cream Cheese and Eggs)

Day 47
- Breakfast: Meat Lover's Breakfast Skillet (Bacon, Sausage, Eggs)
- Starter: Shrimp Cocktail (with Carnivore Sauce)
- Main Dish: Grilled Ribeye Steak with Rosemary Butter
- Side Dish: Buttered Mushrooms
- Dessert: Egg Custard

Day 48
- Breakfast: Bone Broth Breakfast Soup
- Starter: Carnivore Charcuterie Board
- Main Dish: Blackened Catfish

- Side Dish: Cheesy Cauliflower Mash (Carnivore Style)
- Dessert: Cream Cheese Clouds

Day 49

- Breakfast: Smoked Salmon and Scrambled Eggs

Week 8:

Day 50

- Breakfast: Chicken Liver and Eggs
- Starter: Duck Liver Mousse
- Main Dish: Mussels in White Wine Sauce
- Side Dish: Crispy Pork Belly Bites
- Dessert: Beef Tallow Chocolate Fudge

Day 51

- Breakfast: Lamb Kidney and Egg Scramble
- Starter: Carnivore Sushi (Beef and Tuna)
- Main Dish: Sautéed Clams with Bacon
- Side Dish: Parmesan Crusted Zucchini Fries
- Dessert: Whipped Cream with Gelatin

Day 52

- Breakfast: Duck Egg Omelet
- Starter: Bacon-Wrapped Jalapeño Poppers
- Main Dish: Broiled Oysters with Herb Butter
- Side Dish: Pan-Seared Scallops with Bacon
- Dessert: Pork Rind Cookies

Day 53

- Breakfast: Beef Liver and Onion Omelet
- Starter: Salmon Caviar on Egg Slices
- Main Dish: Garlic Shrimp Scampi

Week 9:

Day 57

- Breakfast: Omelet with Cheddar Cheese
- Starter: Chicken Liver Pâté
- Main Dish: Crab Cakes (Carnivore Style)
- Side Dish: Beef Tallow Roasted Brussels Sprouts
- Dessert: Lemon Ricotta Cake

Day 58

- Breakfast: Soft-Boiled Eggs with Sea Salt
- Starter: Pork Rind Nachos
- Main Dish: Blackened Catfish
- Side Dish: Pork Rind Crusted Onion Rings
- Dessert: Salted Caramel Fat Bombs

Day 59

- Breakfast: Egg Muffins with Sausage

- Starter: Grilled Octopus Tentacles
- Main Dish: Shrimp and Crab Boil
- Side Dish: Roasted Bone Marrow
- Dessert: Carnivore Ice Cream (Eggs and Heavy Cream)

- Side Dish: Creamy Spinach (Carnivore Style)
- Dessert: Butter Mousse

Day 54

- Breakfast: Cream Cheese and Egg Puffs
- Starter: Bacon-Wrapped Scallops
- Main Dish: Pan-Seared Scallops with Lemon Butter
- Side Dish: Bacon-Wrapped Jalapeños
- Dessert: Vanilla Egg Pudding

Day 55

- Breakfast: Poached Eggs
- Starter: Beef Tartare
- Main Dish: Grilled Swordfish Steaks
- Side Dish: Carnivore Stuffed Peppers (Ground Meat and Cheese)
- Dessert: Bone Marrow Custard

Day 56

- Breakfast: Scrambled Eggs with Butter
- Starter: Deviled Eggs with Bacon Bits
- Main Dish: Salmon Fillet with Dill Sauce
- Side Dish: Grilled Chicken Skewers
- Dessert: Coconut Oil Chocolate Bars

- Starter: Cheese-Stuffed Mushrooms (Carnivore Version)
- Main Dish: Shrimp and Crab Boil
- Side Dish: Herb Butter Roasted Chicken Wings
- Dessert: Cream Cheese Pancakes

Day 60

- Breakfast: Carnivore Pancakes (Egg and Pork Rinds)
- Starter: Beef Carpaccio
- Main Dish: Mussels in White Wine Sauce
- Side Dish: Sausage and Cheese Stuffed Mushrooms
- Dessert: Bacon and Maple Fat Bombs

Conclusion

Embarking on the carnivore diet is more than just a nutritional change; it's a transformative journey towards optimal health and wellness. Throughout this cookbook, you've discovered the simplicity and power of a meat-centric diet, and hopefully, you've found the recipes both satisfying and invigorating.

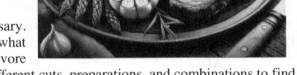

As you continue your carnivore journey, remember that this lifestyle is rooted in the wisdom of our ancestors. By embracing the rich, nutrient-dense foods that have fueled human evolution for millennia, you're giving your body the nourishment it truly craves. The benefits, from improved mental clarity and energy levels to enhanced physical health, are profound and far-reaching.

Cooking and eating should be a joyous experience, and the carnivore diet celebrates that joy in its purest form. The recipes in this book are designed to be not only delicious but also straightforward, making it easy to maintain this way of eating without feeling deprived or overwhelmed.

Always pay attention to your body, and adjust as necessary. Everyone's nutritional needs and responses are unique, and what works for one person might require tweaks for another. The carnivore diet is flexible within its boundaries, allowing you to explore different cuts, preparations, and combinations to find what suits you best.

Made in the USA
Las Vegas, NV
27 September 2024